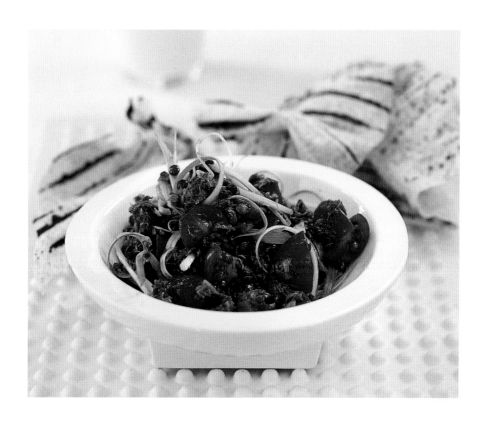

DELICIOUS FOOD FOR DIABETES

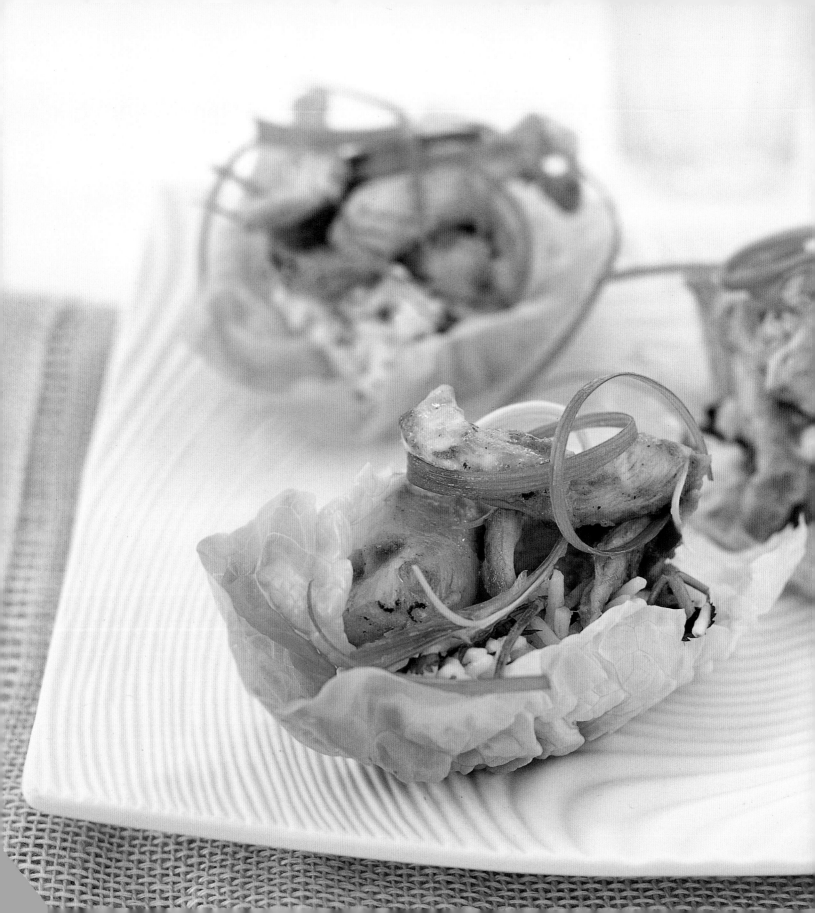

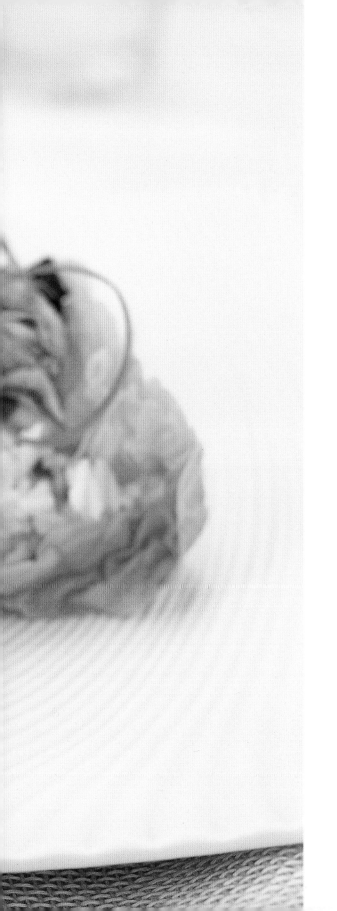

DELICIOUS FOOD FOR DIABETES

OVER 80 TASTY, HEALTHY RECIPES

LOUISE BLAIR

hamlyn

First published in Great Britain in 2005 by
Hamlyn, a division of Octopus Publishing Group Ltd
2–4 Heron Quays, London E14 4JP

ISBN 0 600 61245 7
EAN 9780600612452

A CIP catalogue record for this book is available from the
British Library

Printed and bound in China

10 9 8 7 6 5 4 3 2 1

The publisher has taken all reasonable care in the preparation of this
book, but the information it contains is not intended to take the place
of treatment by a qualified medical practitioner.

Notes
Both metric and imperial measurements are given for the recipes.
Use one set of measures only, not a mixture of both.

Ovens should be preheated to the specified temperature. If using a
fan-assisted oven, follow the manufacturer's instructions for adjusting
the time and temperature. Grills should also be preheated.

This book includes dishes made with nuts and nut derivatives. It is
advisable for those with known allergic reactions to nuts and nut
derivatives and those who may be potentially vulnerable to these
allergies, such as pregnant and nursing mothers, invalids, the elderly,
babies and children, to avoid dishes made with nuts and nut oils. It is
also prudent to check the labels of pre-prepared ingredients for the
possible inclusion of nut derivatives.

Meat and poultry should be cooked thoroughly. To test if poultry is
cooked, pierce the flesh through the thickest part with a skewer or
fork – the juices should run clear, never pink or red.

The nutritional analysis refers to each serving.

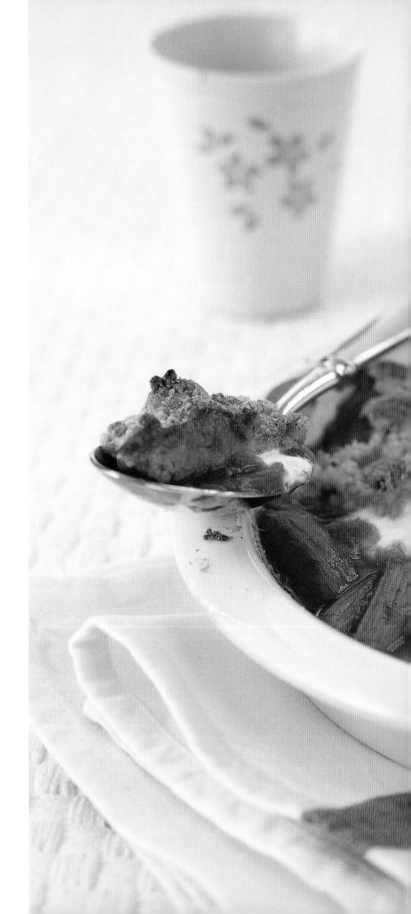

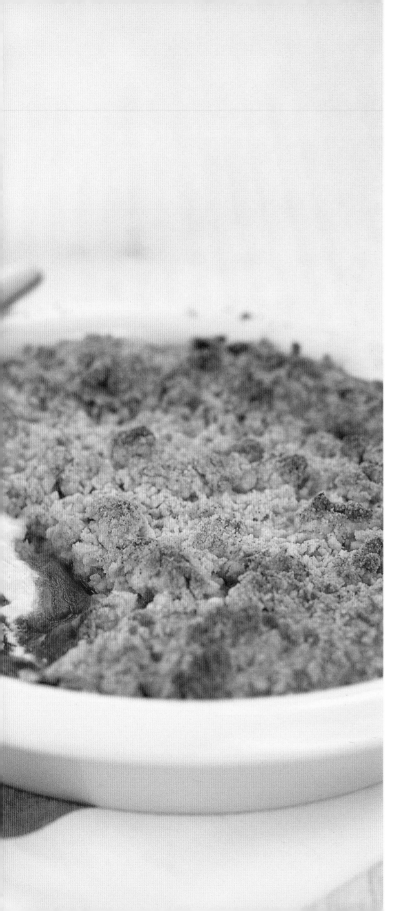

CONTENTS

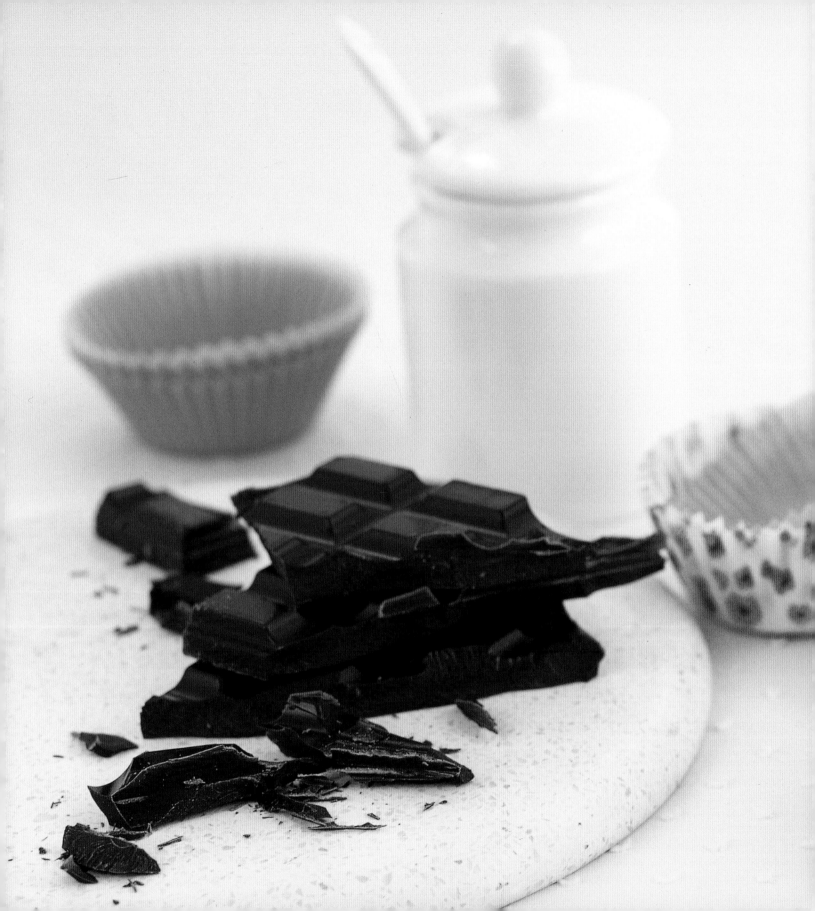

INTRODUCTION

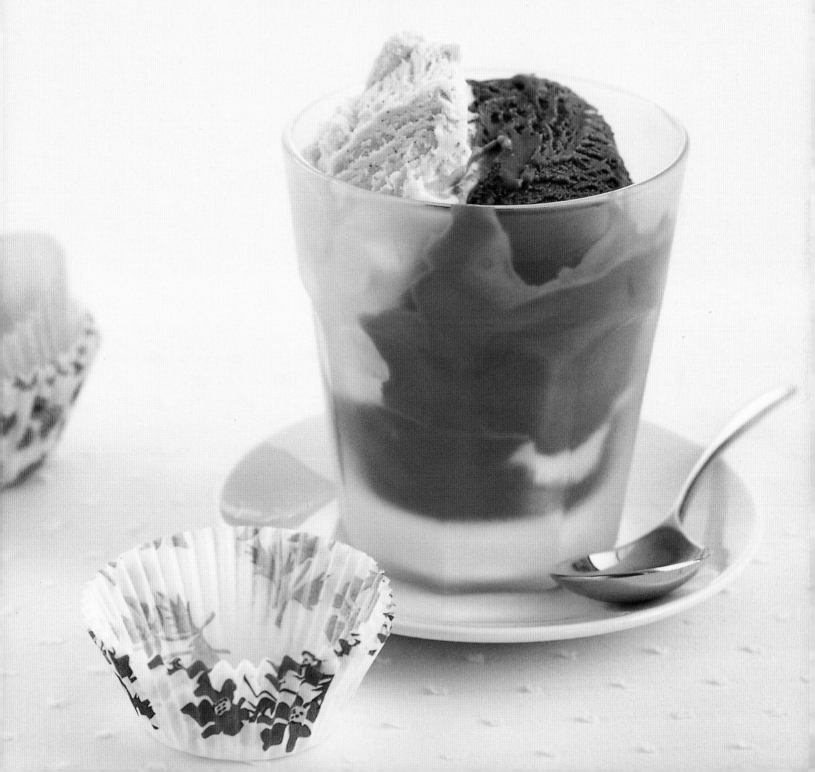

THE DIABETES COOKBOOK

Defining Diabetes

It is estimated that there are up to 1.4 million people with diabetes in the UK alone, mostly with type 2 diabetes. However, there are likely to be about the same number of people who have diabetes without the condition having been diagnosed. The symptoms of diabetes can often mistakenly be put down to other things and it can be years before a routine medical check or a greater awareness of the condition leads individuals to realise they have diabetes. Common symptoms include tiredness, weight loss, a constant thirst and a need to urinate more often than normal.

Diabetes is all to do with a hormone in our bodies called insulin. Insulin acts as a kind of checkpoint for the amount of glucose that is released into the blood and then converted into energy. People with diabetes are either lacking in insulin entirely or it is limited, or their bodies just can't regulate the glucose that's present efficiently. We obtain glucose from various sweet foods such as cakes and biscuits, as well as starchy foods like potatoes, bread and pasta and this glucose is transferred into energy by our bodies. People with diabetes are unable to do this and so the glucose remains unprocessed and stays redundant in the bloodstream. Although it may sound complicated, diabetes is a very treatable condition and, as long as it is recognised and diagnosed quickly, there is no reason for it to result in any long-term health problems.

Types of Diabetes

There are two distinct types of diabetes:

Type 1 diabetes occurs when the body produces no insulin at all. This is also referred to as insulin-dependent diabetes as the treatment for it is a controlled diet and regular insulin injections. It usually develops in younger people and is generally genetic, although it can also be environmental. However, due to the propensity for type 1 diabetes to be genetic, certain individuals will be at higher risk if the condition runs in their family and, if there is a history of diabetes, you should be extra vigilant if any warning signs occur.

Type 2 diabetes occurs when a certain amount of insulin can still be produced by the body but it is not sufficient to transfer glucose into energy effectively. It may also be that insulin is being produced but the body isn't making use of it efficiently. This form of diabetes generally affects older people, though not exclusively. There are different combinations of treatment, depending on the individual – sometimes it can be controlled simply by changes to the diet, regular exercise and tablets. Otherwise, a change in diet may be combined with insulin injections. Type 2 diabetes can develop very slowly and it often goes undetected for years, which is when more serious complications can arise.

Can Anyone Develop Diabetes?

Type 1 diabetes will usually develop when a child is quite young, although it can occur up until the age of about 40. It isn't fully understood why the condition develops but there isn't anything that can be done to avoid this type of diabetes. **Type 2 diabetes** on the other hand can be prevented in some cases, or at the very least diagnosed at the earliest possible opportunity and treated quickly and effectively. Certain people will be more at risk or predisposed to developing type 2 diabetes and these include people of Asian or African-Caribbean origin. Other potential risk groups revolve mainly around life stage and

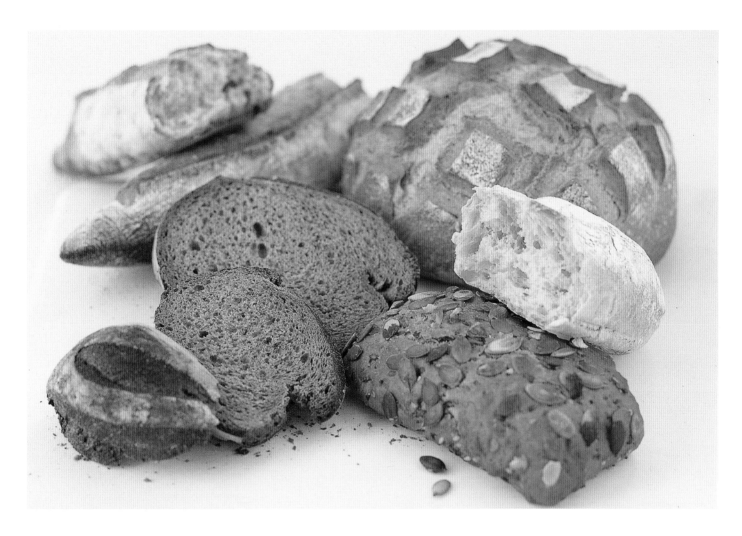

lifestyle; your chances of developing type 2 diabetes will be increased if you are older, if you suffer from obesity or if you don't take sufficient, regular exercise. Recent studies have revealed that people who eat junk food on a regular basis (more than twice a week) are twice as likely to develop type 2 diabetes. This is because of the high fat and salt content and low nutritional value of fast food. In rarer cases, certain medication can increase the risk of diabetes, as can pregnancy or any disease that damages the pancreas and has an impact on its insulin-producing ability.

Dealing with Hypos

People with diabetes need to be extremely in tune with their bodies so they can react quickly if their blood glucose levels fall

Above Wholegrain and brown breads are high in fibre and complex carbohydrates, which are more effective at controlling blood glucose.

suddenly. If you're using insulin or certain kinds of tablets, you must always ensure that you have a snack between meals to avoid such a situation. This is referred to as hypoglycaemia or a 'hypo' and can be dealt with quickly by the individual having a quick-acting sugar, such as a sugary drink, some chocolate, glucose sweets or sugar cubes. This is a quick-fix measure that will stop the immediate effects but should be followed up with a long-lasting carbohydrate such as a bowl of cereal, a piece of toast or a muesli bar. Individuals will come to identify their own hypo symptoms and these will tend to vary but they often include any combination of the following: increased pulse rate,

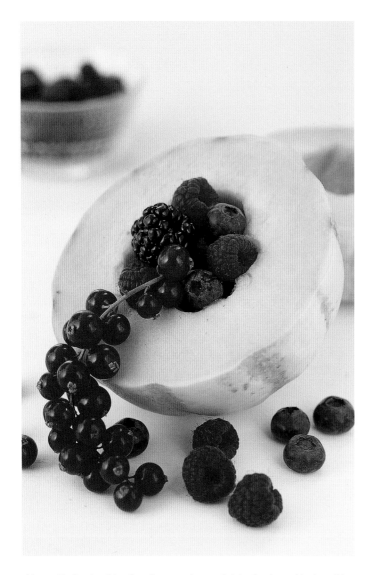

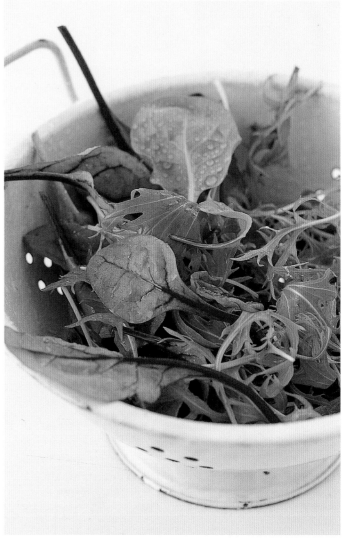

Above Eating healthy day-time snacks needn't be boring with the wide range of delicious fruits that are available.

Above Eating salad with your main meal can help you achieve your five-a-day quota of fruit and vegetables.

shaking, blurred vision, sweating and feeling hungry. Hypos can be the result of a number of things but are typically due to the sufferer missing a meal or eating insufficient carbohydrates. That's why regular meals and suitable snacks are such an important part of diabetes control. A hectic lifestyle often means that meals are delayed for reasons beyond your control but the important thing is to be prepared and treat a hypo as soon as you experience any of the symptoms.

Eating to Control Diabetes

Diet plays a huge role in the control of diabetes and, when combined with exercise and medication (where required), can result in minimal interruptions to the daily lives of people with diabetes. It's really all about taking more of a keen interest in what you eat and ensuring that you eat regularly and sensibly. As this book demonstrates, this doesn't mean a lifetime of boring, repetitive meals. The key to controlling your diabetes is not about switching to a strict, new diet, it's just about eating a generally healthy diet – something that everyone should be aiming to do.

As a basic guideline, all food can be divided into one of five main groups, and to achieve a healthy, well-balanced diet we should aim to eat a certain amount from each group. The five groups are:

Bread, Potatoes and Cereals
Meals should be based around one of these – starchy foods should make up the bulk of your diet as they will fill you up but aren't high in fat.

Fruit and Vegetables
Aim to eat five portions of fruit and vegetables a day. Accompany your main meals with a side salad, and snack on fruit during the day to help achieve this quota.

Milk and Dairy Products
Dairy products are essential for calcium – opt for low-fat varieties wherever possible.

Meat, Fish and Alternatives
This food group includes pulses, beans and soya products. When eating meat, trim off all the visible fat and remove any skin.

Foods containing Fat and/or Sugar
Eat smaller amounts of these types of foods and use oil and butter sparingly. Cakes, biscuits and other processed foods have no nutritional benefits and should be eaten only occasionally as a treat.

Generally speaking, you should ensure you eat regular meals and base them around fruit, vegetables and healthy carbohydrates, in order to regulate your blood glucose levels. Choose wholegrain or brown varieties of bread, pasta and rice,

Right Pulses and beans are an excellent and healthy protein alternative to eating meat.

as these are high in fibre and complex carbohydrates, which take longer to break down and are more effective at controlling blood glucose. By eating a healthier diet and making simple changes, such as switching from full fat to semi-skimmed milk, you should also lose excess weight, which is another important factor in helping to control diabetes. Here are some more guidelines that should be followed to help to control the symptoms of diabetes:

• Eating too much salt can lead to high blood pressure so try and cut down on the amount you eat. If you season food with salt while you're cooking, don't add any more once the meal is served.

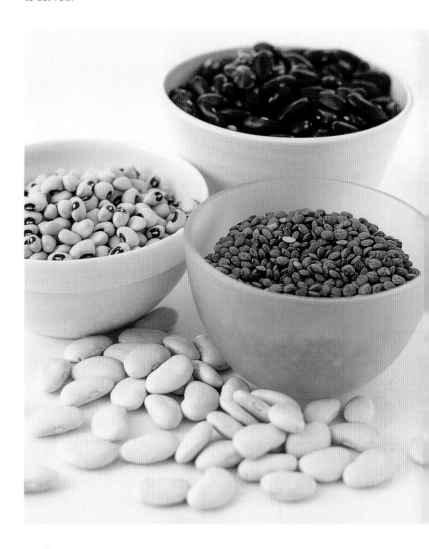

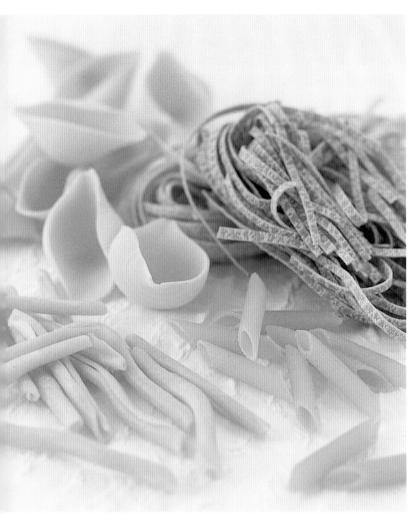

Above There is a huge variety of pastas available today; not only do they help fill you up, but they are fat-free.

• Opt for sugar-free or diet drinks.

• Cut down on the amount of fat in your diet, in particular saturated animal fats. Use a monounsaturated oil, such as olive oil, for cooking and switch to lower fat versions of dairy products, such as skimmed or semi-skimmed milk.

• Limit your alcohol consumption to two units per day for women, or three for men. Roughly speaking one unit is a small glass of wine or half a pint of beer or lager. Avoid drinking alcohol on an empty stomach as this is a major cause of hypoglaecemia. It's particularly important to remember this when going to a party or out for a meal. Have a snack before you go, just to make sure.

• If you are overweight, aim to lose some weight through a combination of dietary changes and regular exercise. Excess weight can be bad for your heart and will affect your blood glucose levels.

• Finally, don't be tempted to buy specific diabetic products or foods. They offer no further benefits than an overall healthy diet and are a waste of money.

The Glycaemic Index

Also referred to as GI, this eating plan has gained considerable popularity in recent years mainly because it isn't especially limiting or restrictive and can be based around your lifestyle. The glycaemic index is a reference number that is applied to all carbohydrate foods and it measures the rate at which that food is broken down into blood glucose and therefore the impact it has on blood glucose levels. It also takes into account the amount of fat, fibre and protein that is present in the food, as these factors will all have an impact on how it is digested and broken down. Put simply, there are two types of carbohydrates: simple and complex and we should be eating more of the complex carbs and reducing our intake of simple or refined carbs. The idea is that you choose a combination of foods that will complement each other and result in a steady blood glucose level that doesn't peak or fluctuate wildly, thus eliminating hunger pangs, mood swings and the desire to tuck into quick-fix foods such as crisps and processed meals. This way of eating ties in well with the guidelines set out for diabetes sufferers and is based around creating balanced meals and snacks that are mainly low or medium GI, combined with a limited intake of high GI foods. So, for example, lentils, porridge oats, granary bread, leafy green vegetables and apples are examples of good choices, while white bread, white rice, crisps, baked potatoes and processed ready-meals are higher-GI foods. If you eat these then try to combine them with low-GI foods to create the right balance.

Embracing A Healthy Lifestyle

Although it's advised that everyone takes regular exercise as part of a healthy lifestyle, this is in fact one of the main ways used to control diabetes and should be taken on board as part of the treatment process. There are many benefits including:

• Regulating glucose levels
• Lowering blood pressure
• Reducing fat around the organs
• Strengthening the heart
• Improving circulation

With diabetes there are extra considerations when it comes to exercise. You will need to adjust your carbohydrate intake depending on the level and endurance of exercise that you're doing and monitor your blood glucose levels before, during and after any activity. This is especially important when you're just starting a new exercise programme. As you progress, you'll learn how your body adapts and copes and should have a better idea of exactly what you need to eat to compensate for any particular activity. Your body will keep on using up energy reserves even after you've finished exercising so it's important to keep an eye on blood sugar levels and have a snack, if necessary. A banana or a couple of handfuls of raisins should be adequate if you're doing a moderate activity; however if you're embarking on strenuous exercise you'll need to increase your carb intake accordingly before and during the activity. For example, you may want to have a bagel beforehand and keep a muesli bar and a sugary drink handy to have while you're exercising, in case of a hypo.

Indulgence and Entertaining

There are a couple of things to remember when you're eating out. If your diabetes is insulin dependent, make sure you keep insulin with you and be extra vigilant about spotting hypo symptoms. Be aware that it might take a little while for food to arrive in a restaurant so you might want to have a discreet sugary snack to hand or otherwise ask for some bread if there

Right Just because you have diabetes, it doesn't mean that you can't enjoy delicious desserts. Try the St Clements Cheesecake on page 124.

isn't any already on the table. Other than that, it's just a case of choosing sensible options from restaurant menus or ensuring that you only indulge in 'bad' foods once in a while.

You can still enjoy eating out and cooking for friends, and there are plenty of ideas in this book for entertaining – impress your guests with impressive dishes such as Goats' Cheese and Herb Soufflés (page 83), followed by Sesame Crusted Salmon with Stir-fried Vegetables (page 90). There are also quick family meals such as Aromatic Chicken Pilaf (page 29), and Chargrilled Lamb with Hummus and Tortillas (page 42), as well as delicious snacks and desserts and quick-cook meals for when you're busy. If people don't know about your diabetes, they certainly won't guess from the meals you prepare!

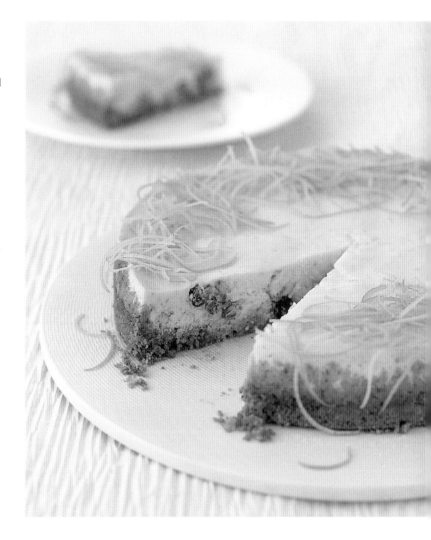

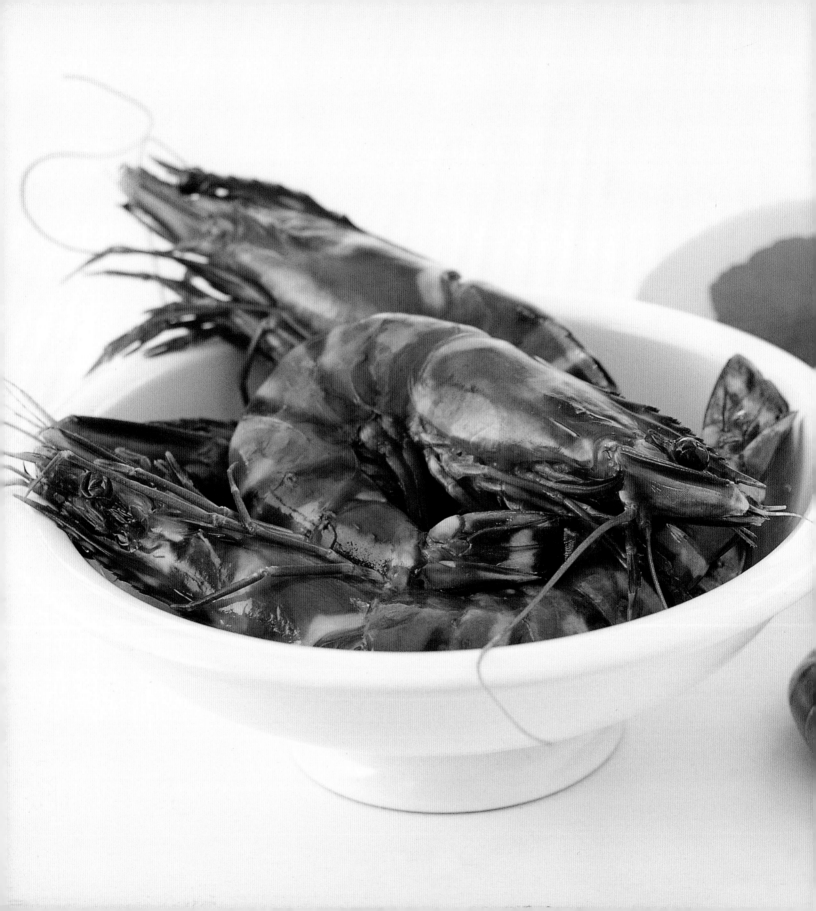

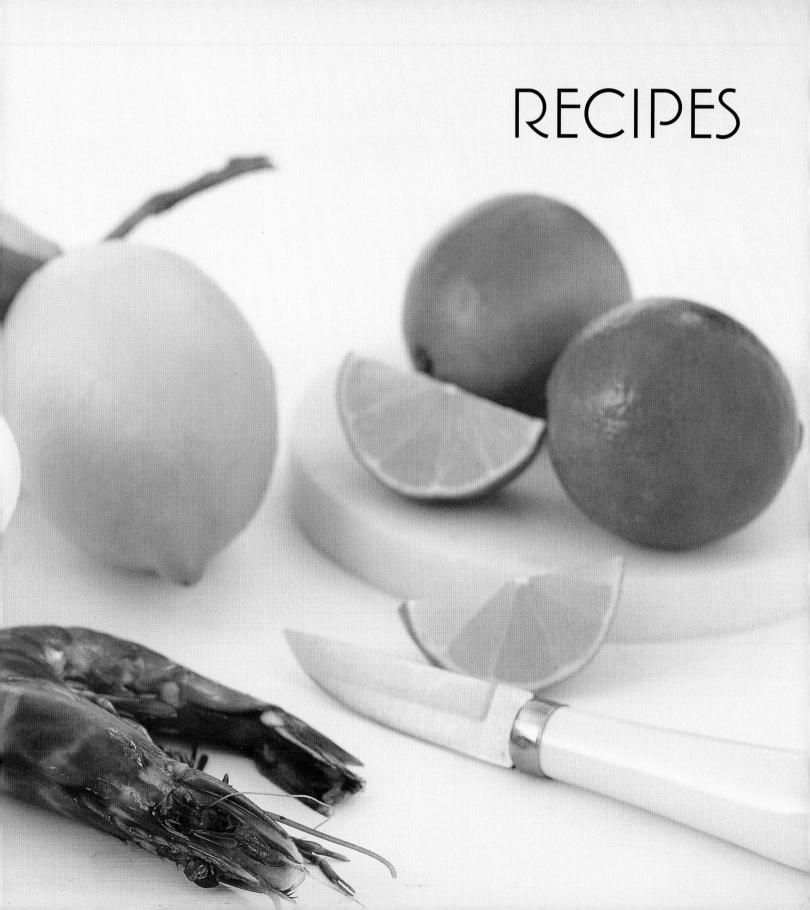

RECIPES

WEEKDAY WONDERS

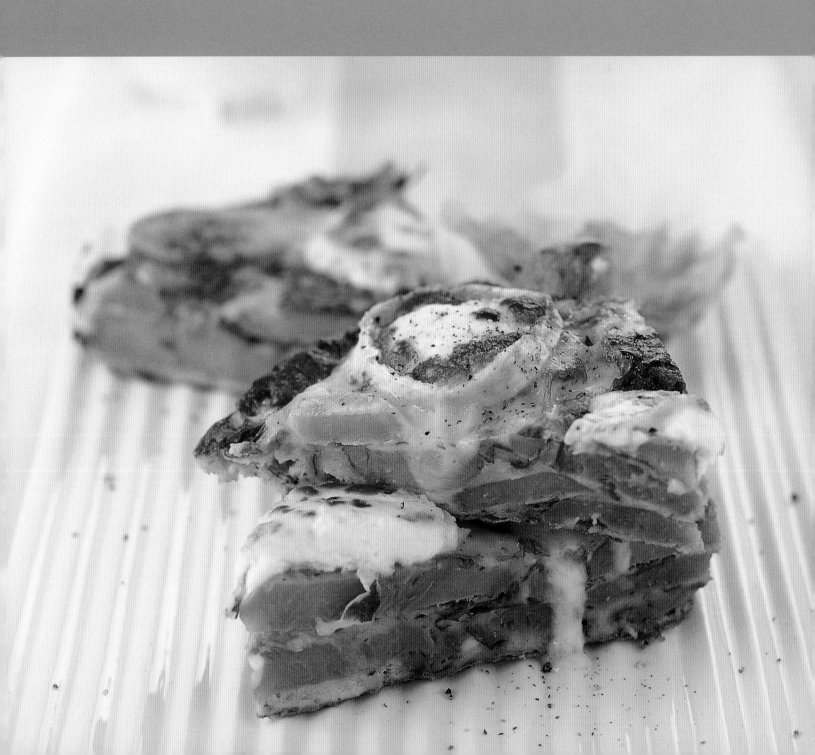

SWEET POTATO, GOATS' CHEESE
AND CORIANDER FRITTATA

serves 4

preparation time 10 minutes

cooking time 20 minutes

nutritional values per serving

Kcals 247 (1020 kj) Protein 12 g Carb 25 g Fat 12 g

Saturated fat 2 g Fibre 2 g

---

500 g (1 lb) sweet potatoes, sliced

1 teaspoon olive oil

5 spring onions, sliced

2 tablespoons chopped coriander

4 large eggs, beaten

1 x 100 g (3½ oz) round goats' cheese with rind, cut into 4 slices

pepper

crisp green salad, to serve

1 Place the sweet potato slices in a saucepan of boiling water and cook for 7–8 minutes until just tender. Drain.

2 Heat the oil in a medium nonstick frying pan, add the spring onions and sweet potato slices and fry for 2 minutes.

3 Stir the coriander into the beaten eggs, season with plenty of pepper and pour into the pan. Arrange the slices of goats' cheese on top and continue to cook for 3–4 minutes until almost set.

4 Place the pan under a high grill and cook for 2–3 minutes until golden and bubbling, then serve with a crisp green salad.

FIERY CHICKEN PIECES
WITH HOT SWEETCORN RELISH

serves 4

preparation time 10 minutes, plus marinating

cooking time 10 minutes

nutritional values per serving

Kcals 466 (1977 kj) Protein 40 g Carb 68 g Fat 7 g

Saturated fat 3 g Fibre 3 g

1–2 green chillies (according to taste), roughly chopped

3 spring onions, chopped

1 garlic clove

2 tablespoons chopped coriander

1 tablespoon sweet chilli sauce

2 teaspoons olive oil

4 boneless, skinless chicken breasts, about 125 g (4 oz) each, sliced

for the relish

1 x 198 g (7 oz) can sweetcorn kernels, drained

125 g (4 oz) cherry tomatoes, chopped

2 spring onions, finely sliced

to serve

4 wholemeal pittas, toasted

4 tablespoons low-fat natural yogurt

1 Place the chillies, spring onions, garlic, coriander, sweet chilli sauce and half the oil in a liquidizer or food processor and blend for a few seconds until combined but still retaining a little texture.

2 Pour over the chicken in a shallow dish and stir well to coat, then cover and leave to marinate in a cool place for 30 minutes.

3 Place the chicken on a baking sheet and cook under a high grill for 5–6 minutes, turning occasionally, until beginning to brown and cooked through.

4 Meanwhile, heat the remaining oil in a frying pan, add the sweetcorn and fry for 2–3 minutes until golden. Add the tomatoes and spring onions and stir the ingredients together, then serve with the chicken and toasted wholemeal pittas, topped with a spoonful of yogurt.

MOUSSAKA
IN MINUTES

serves 4
preparation time 10 minutes
cooking time 35 minutes

nutritional values per serving
Kcals 348 (1437 kj) Protein 27 g Carb 21 g Fat 17 g
Saturated fat 10 g Fibre 3 g

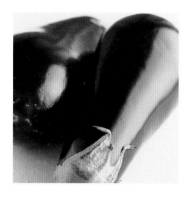

350 g (12 oz) new potatoes

1 teaspoon olive oil

1 large aubergine, chopped

350 g (12 oz) lean minced lamb

1 onion, chopped

400 g (13 oz) can chopped tomatoes

2 tablespoons tomato purée

1 teaspoon chopped oregano

100 g (3½ oz) feta cheese, crumbled

3 tablespoons light Greek yogurt

2 egg yolks, beaten

pepper

Healthy Garlic Bread, to serve (*see page 63*)

1 Place the potatoes in a saucepan of boiling water and cook for 12–15 minutes until tender. Drain, then slice.

2 Meanwhile, heat the oil in a large nonstick frying pan, add the aubergine and fry for 5–6 minutes until just tender. Add the minced lamb and onion and continue to fry for 5 minutes until the lamb is browned.

3 Add the potatoes, tomatoes, tomato purée and oregano and season well with pepper. Bring to the boil and simmer for 15 minutes.

4 Transfer to an ovenproof dish, mix together the feta, yogurt and egg yolks and pour over the mince mixture. Place under a high grill and cook for 3–4 minutes until golden and bubbling. Serve with healthy garlic bread.

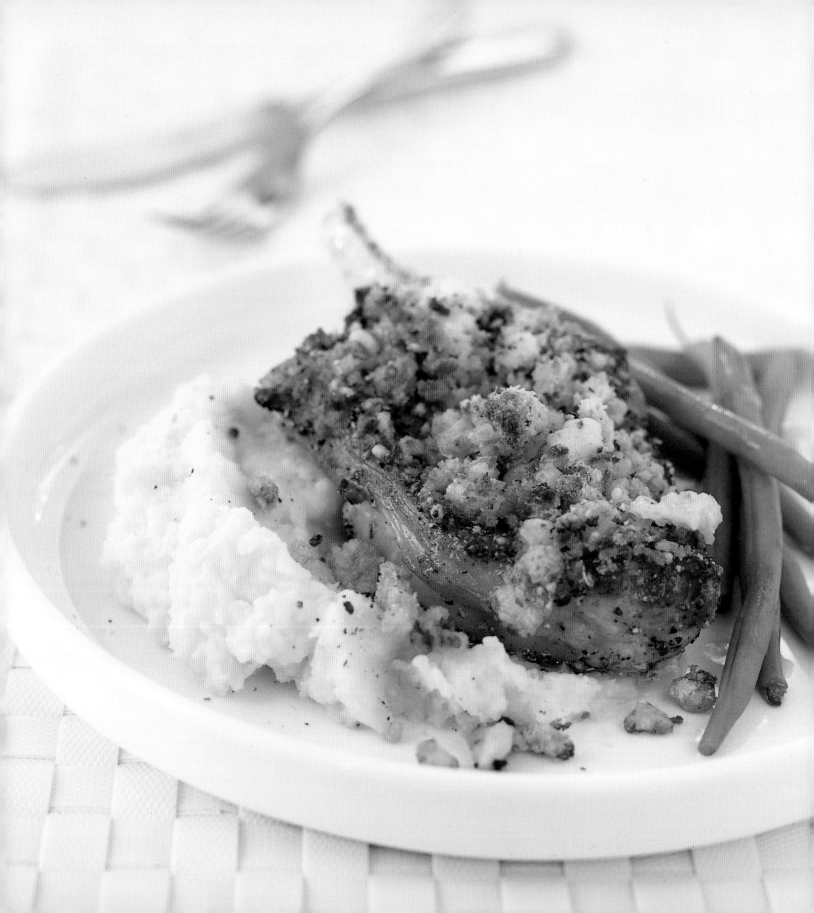

CHEESY HERBED PORK
WITH PARSNIP PURÉE

serves 4

preparation time 10 minutes

cooking time 20 minutes

nutritional values per serving

Kcals 408 (1685 kj) Protein 34 g Carb 29 g Fat 16 g

Saturated fat 7 g Fibre 8 g

---

4 lean pork steaks, about 125 g (4 oz) each

1 teaspoon olive oil

50 g (2 oz) crumbly cheese, e.g., Wensleydale or Cheshire, crumbled

½ tablespoon chopped sage

75 g (3 oz) granary breadcrumbs

1 egg yolk, beaten

steamed green beans or cabbage, to serve

for the parsnip purée

625 g (1½ lb) parsnips, chopped

2 garlic cloves

3 tablespoons light crème fraîche

pepper

1 Season the pork steaks with plenty of pepper. Heat the oil in a nonstick frying pan, add the pork steaks and fry for 2 minutes on each side until browned, then transfer to an ovenproof dish.

2 Mix together the cheese, sage, breadcrumbs and egg yolk. Divide the mixture into 4 and use to top each of the pork steaks, pressing down gently. Cook in a preheated oven, 200°C (400°F), Gas Mark 6, for 12–15 minutes until the topping is golden.

3 Meanwhile, place the parsnips and garlic in a saucepan of boiling water and cook for 10–12 minutes until tender. Drain and mash with the crème fraîche and plenty of pepper, then serve with the pork steaks and some steamed green beans or cabbage.

RATATOUILLE WITH CHICKPEAS

AND SUN-BLUSH TOMATOES

serves 4

preparation time 10 minutes

cooking time 30 minutes

nutritional values per serving

Kcals 394 (1627 kj) Protein 20 g Carb 41 g Fat 16 g

Saturated fat 5 g Fibre 12 g

1 tablespoon olive oil

2 red onions, cut into wedges

2 red peppers, cored, deseeded and cut into chunks

1 orange pepper, cored, deseeded and cut into chunks

1 large aubergine, cubed

3 courgettes, chopped

2 x 400 g (13 oz) cans cherry tomatoes

handful chopped herbs, e.g., parsley, basil, thyme or oregano

50 g (2 oz) sun-blush or sun-dried tomatoes

2 x 400 g (13 oz) cans chickpeas, drained and rinsed

100 g (3½ oz) feta cheese, crumbled

crusty bread, to serve

1 Heat the oil in a large frying pan, add the onions, peppers, aubergine and courgettes and fry for 5–6 minutes until beginning to soften.

2 Add the canned tomatoes and herbs, bring to the boil and simmer for 15 minutes. Add the sun-blush or sun-dried tomatoes and chickpeas and continue to cook for 5 minutes.

3 Top with the feta and serve with a chunk of crusty bread to mop up all the tasty juices.

CREAMY CHICKEN PASTA
WITH LEMON AND PARSLEY

serves 4

preparation time 5 minutes

cooking time 15 minutes

nutritional values per serving

Kcals 383 (1582 kj) Protein 19 g Carb 66 g Fat 6 g

Saturated fat 3 g Fibre 3 g

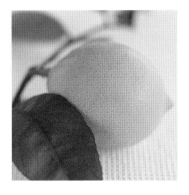

350 g (12 oz) pasta shapes

1 teaspoon olive oil

1 onion, sliced

1 garlic clove, finely sliced

2 large chicken breasts, about 150 g (5 oz) each, cooked and shredded

grated rind and juice of 2 lemons

6 tablespoons light crème fraîche

2 tablespoons chopped parsley

pepper

watercress and rocket salad, to serve

1 Cook the pasta according to the packet instructions. Drain and return to the pan.

2 Meanwhile, heat the oil in a frying pan, add the onion and garlic and fry for 4–5 minutes until softened and beginning to turn golden.

3 Add the remaining ingredients and heat through, then add the drained pasta and toss together. Serve with a watercress and rocket salad.

TUNA-LAYERED LASAGNE
WITH ROCKET

serves 4

preparation time 10 minutes

cooking time 10 minutes

nutritional values per serving

Kcals 210 (867 kj) Protein 22 g Carb 13 g Fat 7 g

Saturated fat 2 g Fibre 3 g

---

8 sheets lasagne

1 teaspoon olive oil

1 bunch spring onions, sliced

2 courgettes, cut into small dice

500 g (1lb) cherry tomatoes, quartered

2 x 200 g (7 oz) cans tuna in water, drained

65 g (2½ oz) rocket

4 teaspoons ready-made pesto

pepper

basil leaves, to garnish

1 Cook the lasagne according to the packet instructions. Drain and return to the pan to keep warm.

2 Meanwhile, heat the oil in a medium frying pan, add the spring onions and courgettes and fry for 3 minutes. Remove from the heat, add the tomatoes, tuna and rocket and gently toss together.

3 Place a little of the tuna mixture on 4 serving plates and top with a sheet of the cooked lasagne. Spoon the remaining tuna mix over the lasagne, then top with the remaining sheets of lasagne. Season with plenty of pepper and top with a spoonful of pesto and some basil leaves before serving.

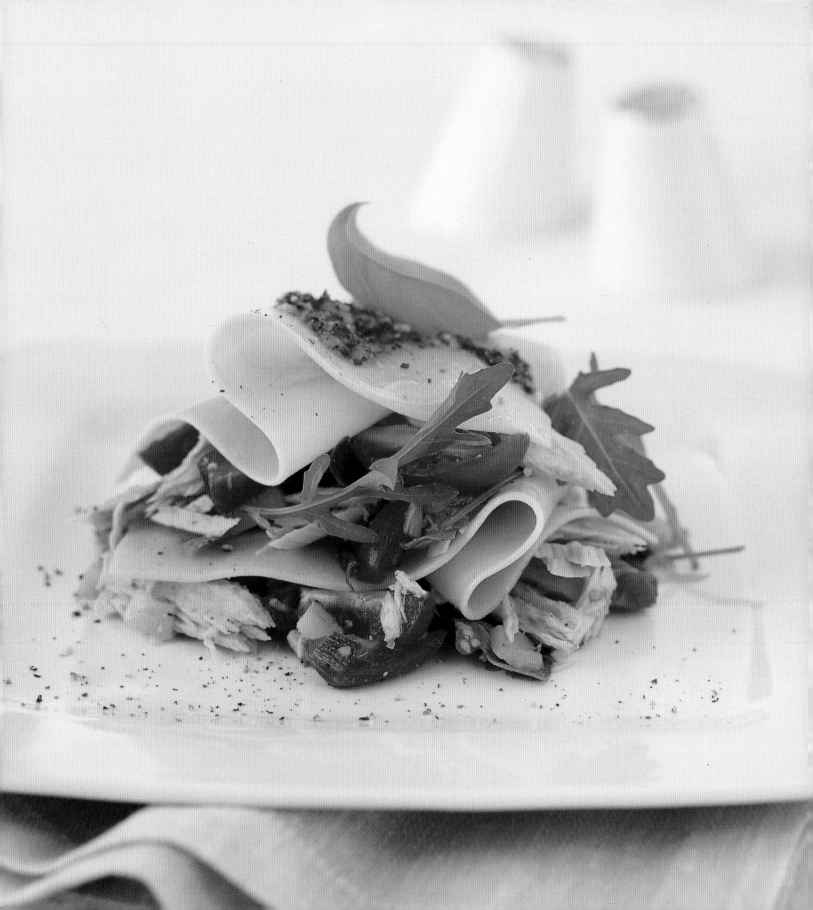

SPAGHETTI

WITH PUTTANESCA SAUCE

serves 4

preparation time 5 minutes

cooking time 15 minutes

nutritional values per serving

Kcals 349 (1441 kj) Protein 12 g Carb 68 g Fat 4 g

Saturated fat 0 g Fibre 4 g

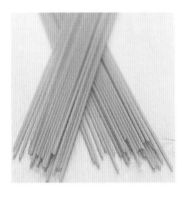

350 g (12 oz) spaghetti

1 teaspoon olive oil

2 garlic cloves, crushed

1 red chilli, finely chopped

4 anchovies, drained and roughly chopped

500 g (1 lb) plum tomatoes, chopped

2 tablespoons capers, drained

40 g (1½ oz) pitted black olives, roughly chopped

3 tablespoons chopped parsley

crisp green salad, to serve

1 Cook the pasta according to the packet instructions. Drain and return to the pan to keep warm.

2 Meanwhile, heat the oil in a nonstick frying pan, add the garlic, chilli and anchovies and fry for 2 minutes.

3 Add the remaining ingredients, except the pasta, bring to the boil and simmer for 5 minutes until the tomatoes are pulpy. Add the pasta and toss together, then serve with a crisp green salad.

CARBONARA

WITH PARMA HAM AND ROCKET

serves 4

preparation time 5 minutes

cooking time 15 minutes

nutritional values per serving

Kcals 438 (1808 kj) Protein 21 g Carb 65 g Fat 11 g

Saturated fat 6 g Fibre 8 g

---

350 g (12 oz) wholemeal spaghetti

100 g (3½ oz) Parma ham, cut into strips

6 tablespoons light crème fraîche

3 tablespoons freshly grated Parmesan cheese

2 egg yolks, beaten

100 g (3½ oz) rocket

pepper

mixed salad leaves, including rocket, to serve

1 Cook the pasta according to the packet instructions. Drain and return to the pan.

2 Add the Parma ham, crème fraîche, Parmesan and egg yolks to the pasta and toss together. Heat for about a minute, over a low heat, until the egg yolks are just cooked.

3 Toss through the rocket and season well with pepper. Serve with mixed salad leaves, including rocket.

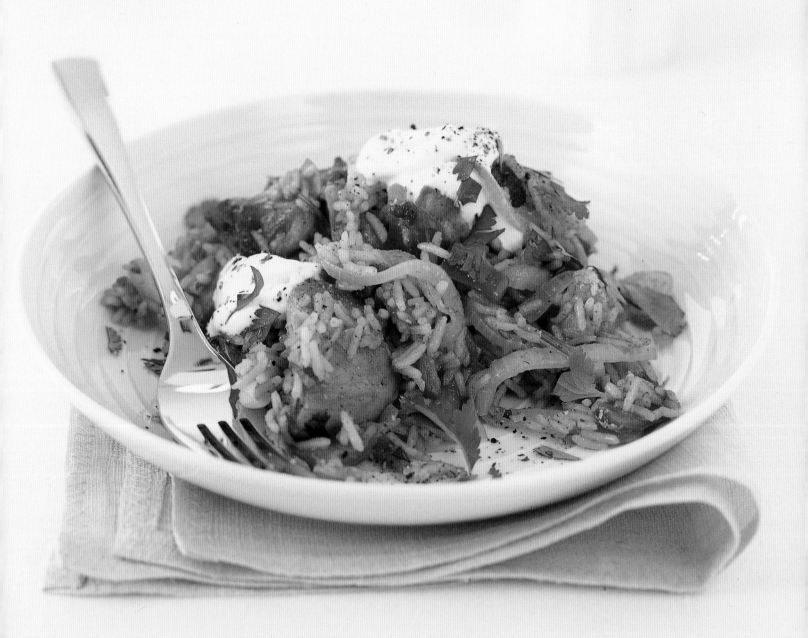

AROMATIC
CHICKEN PILAF

serves 4

preparation time 10 minutes, plus standing

cooking time 25 minutes

nutritional values per serving

Kcals 465 (1920 kj) Protein 30 g Carb 67 g Fat 8 g

Saturated fat 3 g Fibre 3 g

---

1 tablespoon olive oil

1 onion, sliced

1 garlic clove, chopped

1 red pepper, cored, deseeded and chopped

1 teaspoon cumin seeds

1 teaspoon ground coriander

2 teaspoons chilli powder

2 teaspoons curry powder

4 large boneless, skinless chicken thighs, about 100 g (3½ oz) each, cut into bite-sized pieces

200 g (7 oz) basmati rice

600 ml (1 pint) chicken stock (made with concentrated liquid stock)

125 g (4 oz) ready-to-eat dried apricots, chopped

3 tablespoons chopped coriander

4 tablespoons light Greek yogurt

1 Heat the oil in a nonstick frying pan, add the onion, garlic and pepper and fry for 3–4 minutes until softened.

2 Add the spices and continue to fry for 1 minute, then add the chicken and cook for 2 minutes until browned all over. Add the rice to the pan and stir to combine.

3 Stir in the stock and apricots, cover well and simmer for 15 minutes, then leave to stand for 5 minutes.

4 Scatter over the coriander, top each serving with a spoonful of yogurt and serve.

BACON AND TALEGGIO
TORTILLA PIZZAS

serves 4
preparation time 10 minutes
cooking time 25 minutes

nutritional values per serving
Kcals 319 (1317 kj) Protein 20 g Carb 31 g Fat 11 g
Saturated fat 6 g Fibre 1 g

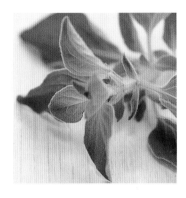

250 g (8 oz) new potatoes
4 flour tortillas
6 tablespoons Tomato Salsa (*see page 35*)
50 g (2 oz) lean bacon, chopped
4 spring onions, sliced
100 g (3½ oz) Taleggio cheese, thinly sliced
1 tablespoon chopped oregano
2 tablespoons light crème fraîche
pepper
green salad, to serve

1 Place the potatoes in a saucepan of boiling water and cook for 12–15 minutes until tender. Drain, then slice.

2 Meanwhile, place the tortillas on baking sheets (you may have to cook these in batches) and spoon over the tomato salsa.

3 Place the bacon in a small nonstick frying pan and fry for 2–3 minutes until browned.

4 Lay the potatoes, spring onions and bacon on the tortillas, then top with the Taleggio and oregano and season well with pepper. Bake in a preheated oven, 220°C (425°F), Gas Mark 7, for 8–10 minutes until golden and bubbling.

5 Spoon over the crème fraîche and serve with a green salad.

Make your own combinations by choosing from some of the following toppings: artichoke hearts, Parma ham, pear, rocket, roasted vegetables, goats' cheese, ricotta cheese, blue cheese, sliced tomato, olives, tuna, sultanas, fried leek. Alternatively, you can invent your own toppings, but try to keep the fat content and calories down by choosing sensibly.

SWEET POTATO, PARSNIP
AND CABBAGE SOUP

serves 4

preparation time 15 minutes

cooking time 25 minutes

nutritional values per serving

Kcals 160 (660 kj) Protein 5 g Carb 35 g Fat 2 g

Saturated fat 1 g Fibre 6 g

---

2 onions, chopped

2 garlic cloves, sliced

4 lean back bacon rashers, chopped

500 g (1 lb) sweet potatoes, chopped

2 parsnips, chopped

1 teaspoon chopped thyme

1 quantity Vegetable Stock (*see page 55*)

1 baby Savoy cabbage, shredded

Irish soda bread, to serve

1 Place the onions, garlic and bacon in a large saucepan and fry for 2–3 minutes.

2 Add the sweet potatoes, parsnips, thyme and stock, bring to the boil and simmer for 15 minutes.

3 Transfer two-thirds of the soup to a liquidizer or food processor and blend until smooth. Return to the pan, add the cabbage and continue to simmer for 5–7 minutes until the cabbage is just cooked. Serve with Irish soda bread.

SMOKED HADDOCK
WITH POACHED EGGS AND CRUSHED POTATOES

serves 4

preparation time 10 minutes

cooking time 30 minutes

nutritional values per serving

Kcals 397 (1639 kj) Protein 47 g Carb 32 g Fat 9 g

Saturated fat 3 g Fibre 2 g

---

750 g (1½ lb) new potatoes

4 spring onions, sliced

2 tablespoons light crème fraîche

75 g (3 oz) watercress

4 smoked haddock fillets, about 150g (5 oz) each

150 ml (¼ pint) semi-skimmed milk

1 bay leaf

4 eggs

pepper

1 Place the potatoes in a saucepan of boiling water and cook for 12–15 minutes until tender. Drain, lightly crush with a fork, then stir through the spring onions, crème fraîche and watercress and season well with pepper. Keep warm.

2 Place the fish and milk in a large frying pan with the bay leaf. Bring to the boil, then cover and simmer for 5–6 minutes until the fish is cooked through.

3 Meanwhile, bring a saucepan of water to the boil, swirl the water with a spoon and crack in an egg, allowing the white to wrap around the yolk. Simmer for 3 minutes, then remove and keep warm. Repeat with the remaining eggs.

4 Serve the haddock on the potatoes, topped with the poached eggs.

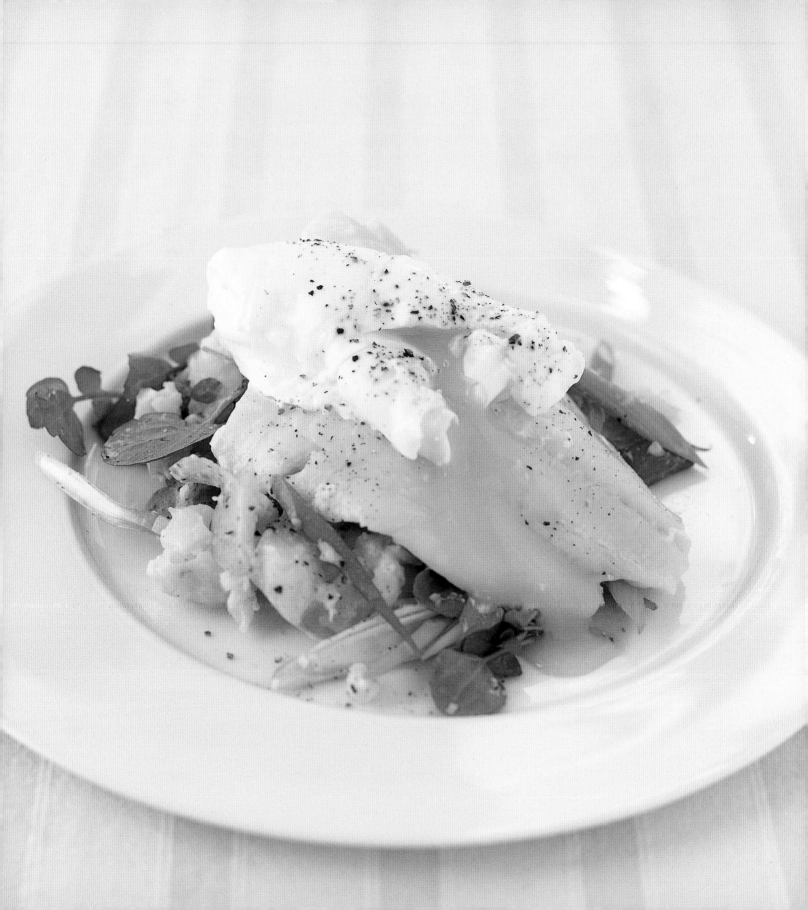

ROASTED PUMPKIN

WITH LAMB AND ONION STUFFING

serves 4

preparation time 10 minutes

cooking time 1¾ hours

nutritional values per serving

Kcals 226 (933 kj) **Protein** 19 g **Carb** 22 g **Fat** 7 g

Saturated fat 4 g Fibre 7 g

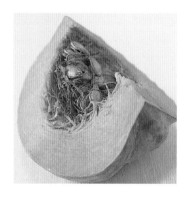

1 pumpkin, about 2 kg (4 lb), or 2 weighing 1 kg (2 lb) each

1 onion, chopped

350 g (12 oz) lean minced lamb

1 cooking apple, peeled, cored and chopped

50 g (2 oz) sultanas

400 g (13 oz) can chopped tomatoes

2 tablespoons tomato purée

few drops Tabasco sauce (optional)

1 tablespoon chopped oregano

pepper

warm bread or rice, to serve

1 Slice the 'lid' off the top of the pumpkin and reserve. Scoop out the seeds with a spoon and discard.

2 Place the onion and minced lamb in a frying pan and fry for 4–5 minutes until browned, then drain off any excess fat. And the remaining ingredients, bring to the boil and simmer for 10 minutes, then season with pepper.

3 Tip the lamb mixture into the hollowed-out pumpkin, replace the lid and cook in a preheated oven, 180°C (350°F), Gas Mark 4, for approximately 1½ hours until the pumpkin is very tender. Scoop out of the shell and serve with warm bread or rice.

CHICKEN BURGERS
WITH TOMATO SALSA

serves 4

preparation time 15 minutes, plus chilling

cooking time 10 minutes

nutritional values per serving

Kcals 135 (558 kj) Protein 20 g Carb 1 g Fat 6 g

Saturated fat 2 g Fibre 1 g

---

1 garlic clove, crushed

3 spring onions, finely sliced

1 tablespoon ready-made pesto

2 tablespoons chopped mixed herbs, e.g., parsley, tarragon, thyme

350 g (12 oz) minced chicken

2 sun-dried tomatoes, finely chopped

1 teaspoon olive oil

for the tomato salsa

250 g (8 oz) cherry tomatoes, quartered

1 red chilli, deseeded and finely chopped

1 tablespoon chopped coriander

grated rind and juice of 1 lime

to serve

4 bread rolls

salad leaves

1 Mix together all the burger ingredients, except the oil. Divide the mixture into 4 and form into burgers. Cover and chill for 30 minutes.

2 Combine all the salsa ingredients in a bowl.

3 Brush the burgers with the oil and cook under a high grill or on a barbecue for about 3–4 minutes each side until cooked through.

4 Serve each burger in a roll with the tomato salsa and salad leaves.

POLENTA-COATED FISH
WITH HOMEMADE CHIPS

serves 4

preparation time 10 minutes

cooking time 30 minutes

nutritional values per serving

Kcals 338 (1396 kj) Protein 34 g Carb 35 g Fat 7 g

Saturated fat 2 g Fibre 2 g

---

750 g (1½ lb) potatoes, cut into thick chips

1 tablespoon olive oil

100 g (3½ oz) polenta

2 tablespoons chopped parsley

1 garlic clove, crushed

grated rind of 1 lemon

4 chunky, skinless white fish fillets, e.g., haddock or cod, about 150 g (5 oz) each

2 eggs, beaten

pepper

mushy peas, to serve

1 Place the potatoes in a saucepan of boiling water and cook for 5 minutes, then drain. Place in a roasting tin and drizzle over a little of the oil, then cook in a preheated oven, 200°C (400°F), Gas Mark 6, for 25–30 minutes until golden.

2 Meanwhile, mix together the polenta, parsley, garlic, lemon rind and plenty of pepper in a shallow dish. Dip each piece of fish into the beaten egg and then into the polenta mixture.

3 Heat the remaining oil in a nonstick frying pan, add the fish and fry for 2–3 minutes on each side until cooked through.

4 Serve with the chips and some mushy peas for a great twist on a usually unhealthy family favourite.

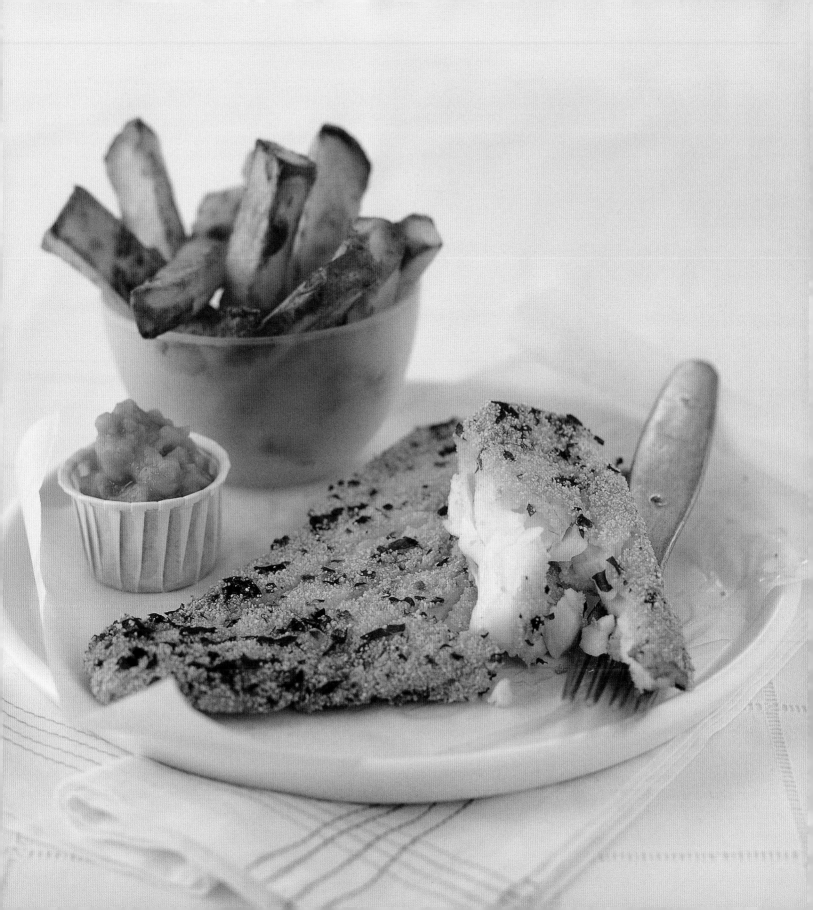

CRAB AND NOODLE

ASIAN WRAPS

serves 4

preparation time 15 minutes, plus standing

cooking time 5 minutes

nutritional values per serving

Kcals 199 (822 kj) Protein 17 g Carb 20 g Fat 5 g

Saturated fat 0 g Fibre 0 g

200 g (7 oz) rice noodles

1 bunch spring onions, finely sliced

1.5 cm (¾ in) piece fresh root ginger, grated

1 garlic clove, finely sliced

1 red chilli, finely chopped

2 tablespoons chopped coriander

1 tablespoon chopped mint

¼ cucumber, cut into fine matchsticks

2 x 175 g (6 oz) cans crabmeat, drained, or 300 g (10 oz) fresh white crabmeat

1 tablespoon sesame oil

1 tablespoon sweet chilli sauce

1 teaspoon Thai fish sauce

16 Chinese pancakes or Vietnamese ricepaper wrappers

1 Cook the rice noodles according to the packet instructions. Drain, then refresh under cold running water.

2 Mix together all the ingredients, except the pancakes or ricepaper wrappers, in a large bowl. Add the noodles and toss to mix. Cover and set aside for 10 minutes to allow the flavours to develop, then transfer to a serving dish.

3 To serve, let people take a pancake or ricepaper wrapper, top with some of the crab and noodle mixture, roll up and enjoy.

You could substitute the crabmeat with vegetables such as peppers and bean sprouts or with cooked pork or minced chicken.

CREAMY BEEF

AND MIXED MUSHROOM STIR-FRY

serves 4

preparation time 5 minutes, plus soaking

cooking time 15 minutes

nutritional values per serving

Kcals 177 (731 kj) Protein 24 g Carb 2 g Fat 8 g

Saturated fat 3 g Fibre 1 g

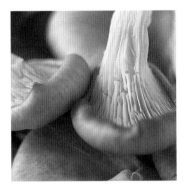

15 g (½ oz) dried porcini mushrooms

150 ml (¼ pint) boiling water

2 teaspoons olive oil

2 onions, sliced

250 g (8 oz) mixed fresh mushrooms, sliced

500 g (1 lb) frying steak, cut into thin strips

4 tablespoons light crème fraîche

1 teaspoon creamed horseradish

1 tablespoon chopped parsley

to serve

brown rice

vegetables

1 Soak the dried mushrooms in the measurement water for 20 minutes. Remove from the soaking liquid, reserving the liquid, and roughly chop.

2 Heat the oil in a nonstick frying pan, add the onions and fry for 3 minutes, then add the fresh mushrooms and continue to fry for 3–4 minutes until cooked.

3 Push the mushroom mixture to one side, add the beef and fry for 3–4 minutes until browned.

4 Pour in the soaking liquid and the dried mushrooms and simmer for 1 minute, then stir in the crème fraîche, horseradish and parsley. Heat through and serve with brown rice and vegetables of your choice.

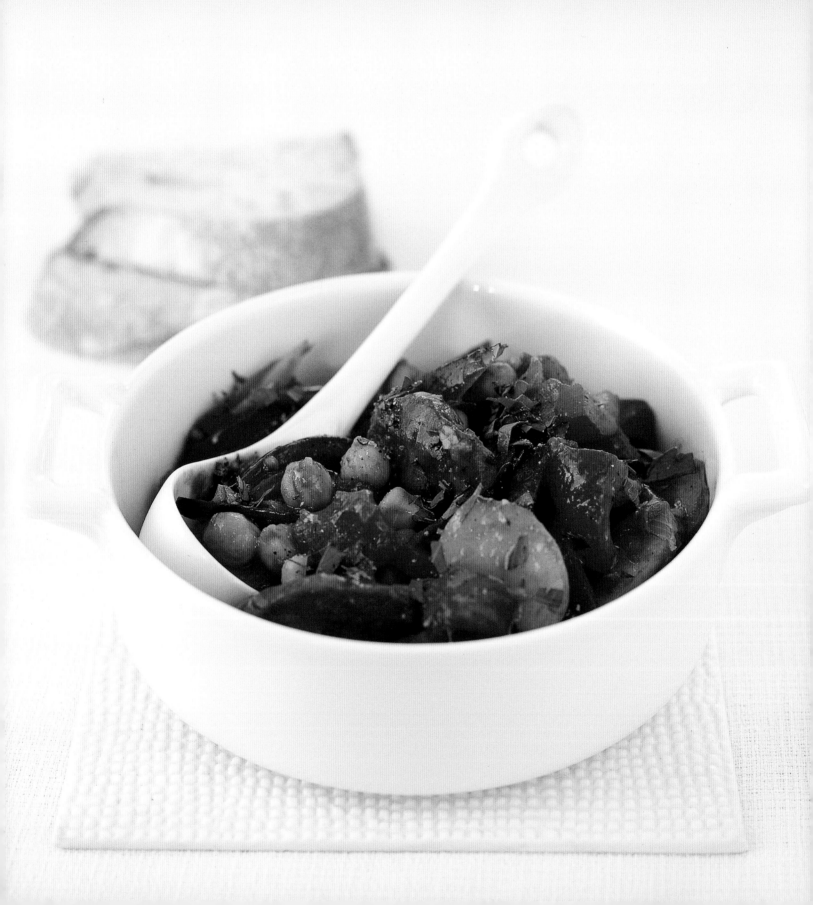

CHORIZO, CHICKPEA
AND RED PEPPER STEW

serves 4

preparation time 5 minutes

cooking time 25 minutes

nutritional values per serving

Kcals 369 (1524 kj) Protein 14 g Carb 45 g Fat 15 g

Saturated fat 1 g Fibre 8 g

---

500 g (1 lb) new potatoes

1 teaspoon olive oil

2 red onions, chopped

2 red peppers, cored, deseeded and chopped

100 g (3½ oz) chorizo sausage, thinly sliced

500 g (1 lb) plum tomatoes, chopped, or a 400 g (13 oz) can tomatoes, drained

400 g (13 oz) can chickpeas, drained and rinsed

2 tablespoons chopped parsley

crusty bread, to serve

1 Place the potatoes in a saucepan of boiling water and cook for 12–15 minutes until tender. Drain, then slice.

2 Meanwhile, heat the oil in a large frying pan, add the onions and peppers and fry for 3–4 minutes until beginning to soften. Add the chorizo and continue to fry for 2 minutes.

3 Add the potato slices, tomatoes and chickpeas, bring to the boil and simmer for 10 minutes. Scatter over the parsley and serve with some crusty bread to mop up all the juices.

CHARGRILLED LAMB
WITH HUMMUS AND TORTILLAS

serves 4

preparation time 10 minutes, plus marinating

cooking time 10 minutes

nutritional values per serving

Kcals 433 (1788 kj) Protein 35 g Carb 44 g Fat 14 g

Saturated fat 6 g Fibre 7 g

---

500 g (1 lb) fillet of lamb, cut into 1.5-cm (¾-in) thick slices

grated rind and juice of 1 lemon

1 rosemary sprig, chopped

3 mixed peppers, cored, deseeded and chopped

1 small aubergine, sliced

4 flour tortillas

rocket, to serve

for the hummus

400 g (13 oz) can chickpeas, drained and rinsed

2 tablespoons light Greek yogurt

2 tablespoons lemon juice

1 tablespoon chopped parsley

1 Place the lamb, lemon rind and juice, rosemary and peppers in a non-metallic bowl and stir well. Cover and leave to marinate in a cool place for 30 minutes.

2 Meanwhile, place the hummus ingredients in a liquidizer or food processor and blend for 30 seconds, then spoon into a bowl.

3 Heat a griddle or heavy-based frying pan until very hot, add the lamb and pepper mixture and the aubergine and fry for 3–4 minutes until cooked. You may need to do this in batches.

4 Meanwhile, heat the tortillas according to the packet instructions. When the lamb and vegetables are ready, wrap in the tortillas with the hummus and serve with some rocket.

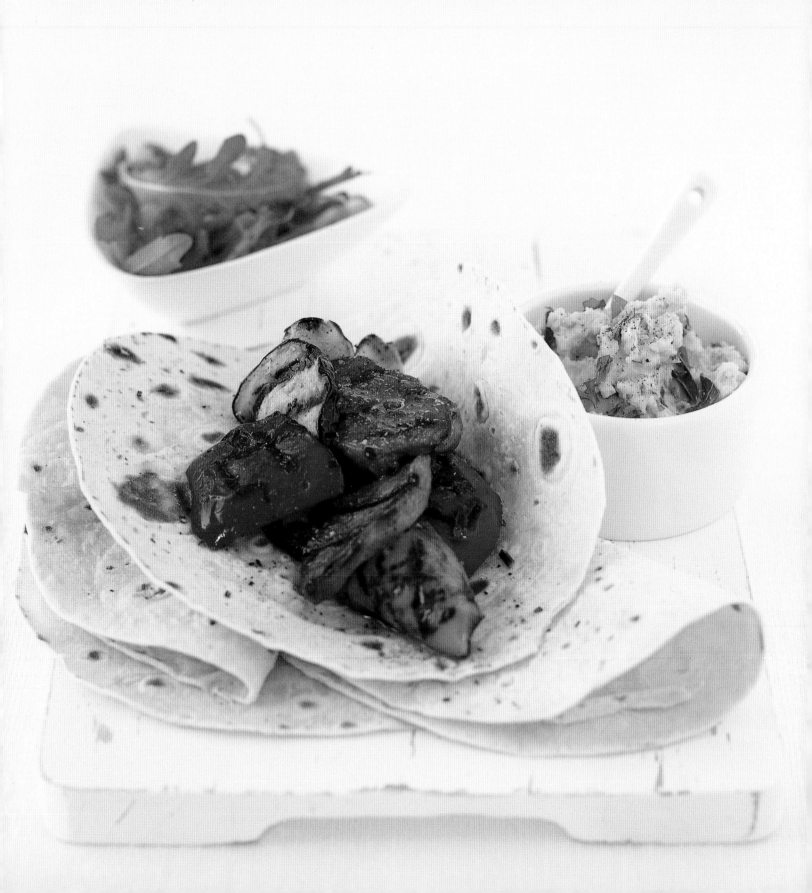

MONKFISH TIKKA
WITH PITTAS

serves 4

preparation time 5 minutes, plus marinating

cooking time 6 minutes

nutritional values per serving

Kcals 389 (1607 kj) Protein 31 g Carb 48 g Fat 9 g

Saturated fat 2 g Fibre 2 g

---

200 ml (7 fl oz) light Greek yogurt

3 tablespoons tikka curry paste

500 g (1 lb) monkfish tail, cut into chunks

4 pittas, toasted

mixed salad leaves, to serve

1 Mix together the yogurt and curry paste in a medium bowl, add the fish and stir well. Cover and leave to marinate in the refrigerator for at least 30 minutes.

2 Place the monkfish pieces on a foil-lined baking sheet and cook under a high grill for 5–6 minutes, turning occasionally, until cooked through.

3 Stuff the pittas with the fish and serve with mixed salad leaves.

COURGETTE, SWEETCORN
AND STILTON FRITTERS

makes 20
preparation time 10 minutes
cooking time 10 minutes

nutritional values per fritter
Kcals 95 (392 kj) Protein 4 g Carb 11 g Fat 3 g
Saturated fat 2 g Fibre 1 g

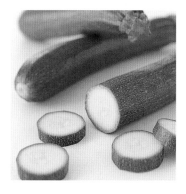

1 tablespoon olive oil

1 large courgette, chopped

3 eggs

150 ml (¼ pint) semi-skimmed milk

150 g (5 oz) self-raising flour, sifted

400 g (13 oz) can flageolet beans, drained and rinsed

handful of parsley, chopped

3 spring onions, sliced

326 g (11 oz) can sweetcorn kernels, drained

100 g (3½ oz) Stilton cheese, crumbled

Tomato Salsa *(see page 35)*, to serve

1 Heat a little of the oil in a nonstick frying pan, add the courgette and fry for 3–4 minutes until golden and tender.

2 Beat together the eggs, milk and flour in a bowl, then stir in the beans, parsley, spring onions, sweetcorn, Stilton and the cooked courgette.

3 Heat the remaining oil in a nonstick frying pan and add tablespoons of the mixture to the pan. Gently flatten each fritter with the back of a fork and fry for 1–2 minutes on each side until golden. Repeat with the remaining mixture, keeping the fritters warm in a low oven.

4 When all the fritters are cooked, serve with tomato salsa.

LIGHT LUNCHES

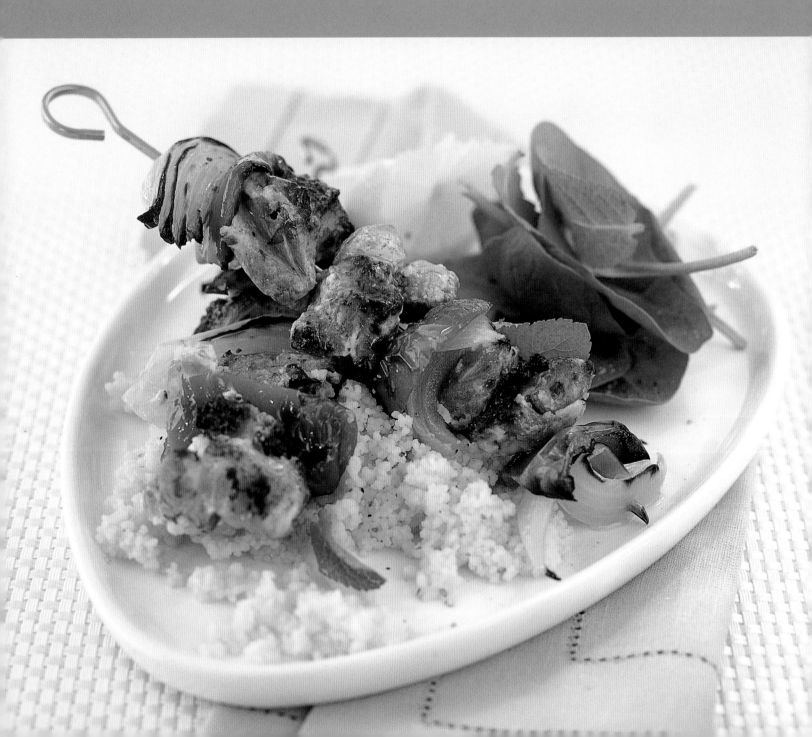

MARINATED MINTY
LAMB KEBABS

serves 4

preparation time 5 minutes, plus marinating

cooking time 10 minutes

nutritional values per serving

Kcals 186 (686 kj) Protein 21 g Carb 8 g Fat 8 g

Saturated fat 4 g Fibre 1 g

---

1 garlic clove, crushed

2 tablespoons chopped mint

1 tablespoon ready-made mint sauce

150 g (5 oz) low-fat natural yogurt

350 g (12 oz) lean lamb, cubed

2 small onions, cut into wedges

1 green pepper, cored, deseeded and cut into wedges

to serve

green salad

couscous

lemon wedges (optional)

1 Mix together the garlic, mint, mint sauce and yogurt in a medium bowl, add the lamb and stir well. Cover and leave to marinate in a cool place for 10 minutes.

2 Thread the lamb and onion and pepper wedges on to 8 metal skewers and cook under a high grill for 8–10 minutes until cooked through. Serve with green salad, couscous and lemon wedges, if desired.

MEDITERRANEAN

STUFFED LOAF

serves 4

preparation time 10 minutes, plus standing

cooking time no cooking

nutritional values per serving

Kcals 364 (1535 kj) Protein 20 g Carb 45 g Fat 13 g

Saturated fat 6 g Fibre 1 g

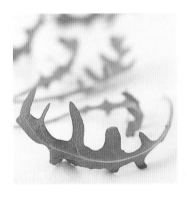

1 medium round loaf, e.g., a boule

2 tablespoons ready-made pesto

75 g (3 oz) rocket

3 plum tomatoes, sliced

75 g (3 oz) Parma ham

400 g (13 oz) can artichoke hearts, drained, rinsed and halved

125 g (4 oz) feta cheese, crumbled

1 Slice a 'lid' off the top of the loaf and reserve. Scoop out most of the bread from the loaf. (This can be made into breadcrumbs and dried or frozen for another day.)

2 Spread the pesto over the insides and base of the hollowed-out loaf, including the lid.

3 Layer the remaining ingredients into the loaf, replace the lid, then wrap in foil or a clean tea towel. Place some dinner plates on top and leave to stand in a cool place for at least 30 minutes. (If you are using this the next day, then store in the refrigerator.)

4 Cut into wedges and serve.

PAN-FRIED CHICKEN LIVERS
WITH BRIOCHE

serves 4

preparation time 10 minutes

cooking time 5 minutes

nutritional values per serving

Kcals 226 (933 kj) Protein 17 g Carb 21 g Fat 8 g

Saturated fat 2 g Fibre 1 g

---

1 tablespoon olive oil

2 spring onions, sliced

250 g (8 oz) chicken livers

8 canned artichoke hearts, drained, rinsed and halved

1 tablespoon chopped sage

1 tablespoon balsamic vinegar

4 brioche rolls, halved and toasted

1 Heat the oil in a nonstick frying pan, add the spring onions and chicken livers and fry for 2–3 minutes until the livers are just cooked.

2 Add the artichoke hearts, sage and balsamic vinegar, mix together and heat through. Serve with the toasted brioche rolls.

RYE SANDWICH

WITH LEMON TARRAGON CHICKEN

serves 4

preparation time 10 minutes

cooking time no cooking

nutritional values per serving

Kcals 228 (942 kj) Protein 20 g Carb 30 g Fat 4 g

Saturated fat 2 g Fibre 4 g

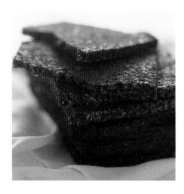

1 Mix together all the ingredients, except the bread, in a medium bowl.

2 Divide the mixture between 4 slices of the bread, then top with the remaining 4 slices, halve and serve.

3 tablespoons light crème fraîche

grated rind and juice of 1 lemon

1 tablespoon chopped tarragon

8 ready-to-eat dried apricots, sliced

2 cooked boneless, skinless chicken breasts, about 150 g (5 oz) each, shredded

large handful of rocket

8 slices rye bread

ROASTED CHERRY TOMATOES
ON CHUNKY TOAST

serves 4

preparation time 5 minutes

cooking time 30 minutes

nutritional values per serving

Kcals 282 (1165 kj) Protein 12 g Carb 38 g Fat 9 g

Saturated fat 2 g Fibre 5 g

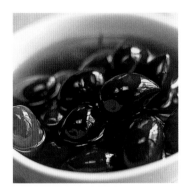

750 g (1½ lb) cherry or plum tomatoes

1 garlic clove, finely chopped

1 tablespoon olive oil

12 black olives

handful of basil, torn

4 thick slices nutty seeded loaf or soda bread, toasted

2 tablespoons fresh Parmesan cheese shavings

pepper

1 Place the tomatoes on a baking sheet, sprinkle over the garlic and oil and cook in a preheated oven, 200˚C (400˚F), Gas Mark 6, for 25–30 minutes until softened.

2 Combine the olives and basil with the tomatoes in a medium bowl and gently toss together along with plenty of pepper.

3 Serve on the slices of toast with the Parmesan shavings sprinkled over the top.

PRAWN, MANGO

AND AVOCADO WRAP

serves 4

preparation time 10 minutes, plus standing

cooking time no cooking

nutritional values per serving

Kcals 311 (1284 kj) Protein 22 g Carb 35 g Fat 10 g

Saturated fat 2 g Fibre 3 g

---

2 tablespoons light crème fraîche

2 teaspoons tomato ketchup

few drops Tabasco sauce

300 g (10 oz) cooked peeled prawns

1 mango, peeled, stoned and thinly sliced

1 avocado, peeled, stoned and sliced

100 g (3½ oz) watercress

4 flour tortillas

1 Mix together the crème fraîche, ketchup and Tabasco to taste in a medium bowl.

2 Add the prawns, mango and avocado and toss the mixture together.

3 Divide the mixture and the watercress between the tortillas, then simply roll up and serve.

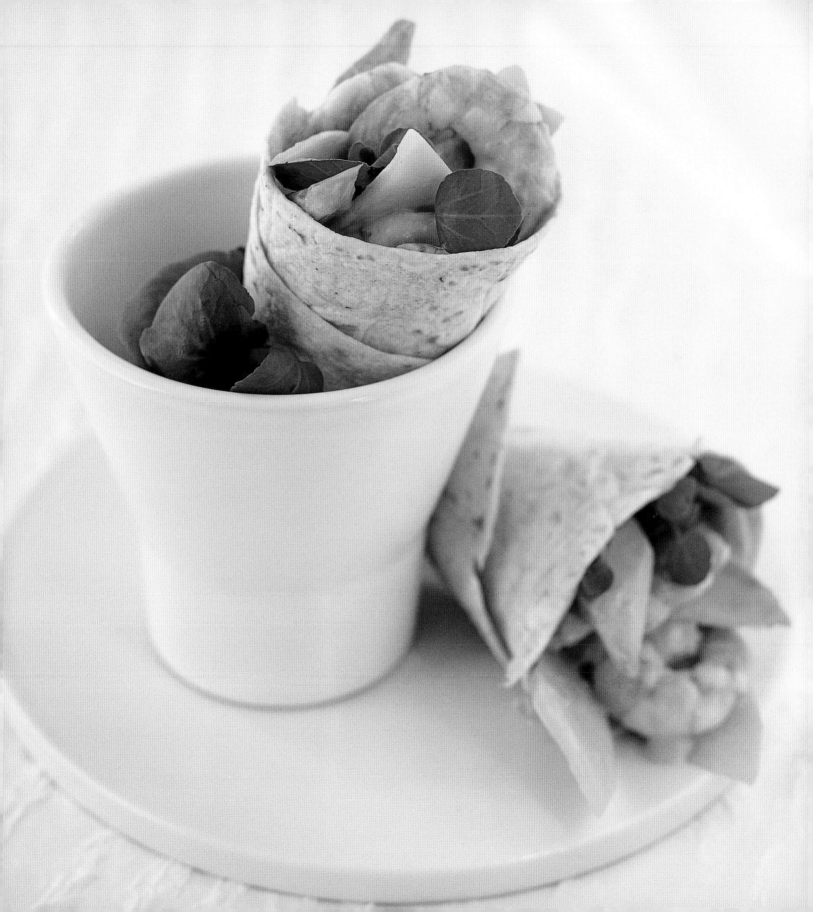

SWEET AND SAVOURY
STUFFED BAGELS

serves 4

preparation time 5 minutes

cooking time no cooking

nutritional values per serving

Kcals 330/341/410 (1363/1408/1693 kj) Protein 24/14/12 g

Carb 47/44/59 g Fat 10/17/18 g

Saturated fat 1/5/6 g Fibre 1/1/1 g

---

4 bagels, halved

for the pastrami and cornichon filling

100 g (3½ oz) pastrami

4 cornichons, sliced

1 small onion, very thinly sliced

2 tablespoons fat-free mayonnaise

1 teaspoon chopped dill

for the cheese 'n' nut filling

100 g (3½ oz) Brie cheese, sliced

25 g (1 oz) walnuts, toasted and roughly chopped

50 g (2 oz) grapes, halved

handful of rocket

for the creamy fruit filling

75 g (3 oz) light cream cheese

4 teaspoons raspberry jam

100 g (3½ oz) mixed berries, e.g., raspberries and sliced strawberries, or 2 nectarines, stoned and sliced

Pastrami and cornichon

1 Layer the pastrami, cornichons and onion on to the bottom halves of the bagels.

2 Mix together the mayonnaise and dill, spoon over the filling, then cover with the top halves of the bagels and serve.

Cheese 'n' nut

1 Divide the ingredients between the bottom halves of the bagels.

2 Cover with the top halves of the bagels and serve.

Creamy fruit

1 Spread the cream cheese and jam over the bottom halves of the bagel and top with the fruit.

2 Cover with the top halves of the bagels and serve.

LENTIL AND PEA SOUP
WITH MINTY CRÈME FRAÎCHE

serves 4

preparation time 10 minutes

cooking time 2 hours

nutritional values per serving

Kcals 141 (582 kj) Protein 11 g Carb 20 g Fat 3 g

Saturated fat 1 g Fibre 6 g

for the vegetable stock

1 tablespoon olive oil

1 onion, chopped

1 carrot, chopped

4 celery sticks, chopped

any vegetable trimmings, such as celery tops, onion skins and tomato skins

1 bouquet garni

1.3 litres (2¼ pints) water

salt and pepper

for the soup

1 teaspoon olive oil

1 leek, finely sliced

1 garlic clove, crushed

400 g (13 oz) can Puy lentils, drained

2 tablespoons chopped mixed herbs, such as thyme and parsley

200 g (7 oz) frozen peas

2 tablespoons light crème fraîche

1 tablespoon chopped mint

pepper

1 To make the stock, heat the oil in a large saucepan, add the vegetables and fry for 2–3 minutes, then add the vegetable trimmings and bouquet garni and season well.

2 Pour over the measurement water, bring to the boil and simmer gently for 1½ hours, by which time the stock should have reduced to 900 ml (1½ pints). Drain over a bowl, discarding the vegetables and retaining the stock.

3 To make the soup, heat the oil in a medium saucepan, add the leek and garlic and fry over a gentle heat for 5–6 minutes until the leek is softened.

4 Add the lentils, stock and herbs, bring to the boil and simmer for 10 minutes. Add the peas and continue to cook for 5 minutes.

5 Transfer half the soup to a liquidizer or food processor and blend until smooth. Return to the pan, stir to combine with the unblended soup, then heat through and season with plenty of pepper.

6 Stir together the crème fraîche and mint and serve on the soup.

QUICK AND EASY

MISO SOUP

serves 4

preparation time 10 minutes

cooking time 1 hour 40 minutes (including
making the stock)

nutritional values per serving

Kcals 56 (231 kj) Protein 6 g Carb 2 g Fat 3 g

Saturated fat 0 g Fibre 0 g

---

1 quantity Vegetable Stock (*see page 55*)

2 tablespoons miso paste

125 g (4 oz) shiitake mushrooms, sliced

200 g (7 oz) tofu, cubed

fresh bread, to serve

1 Place the stock in a saucepan and heat until simmering.

2 Add the miso paste, shiitake mushrooms and tofu to the stock and simmer gently for 5 minutes. Serve with bread.

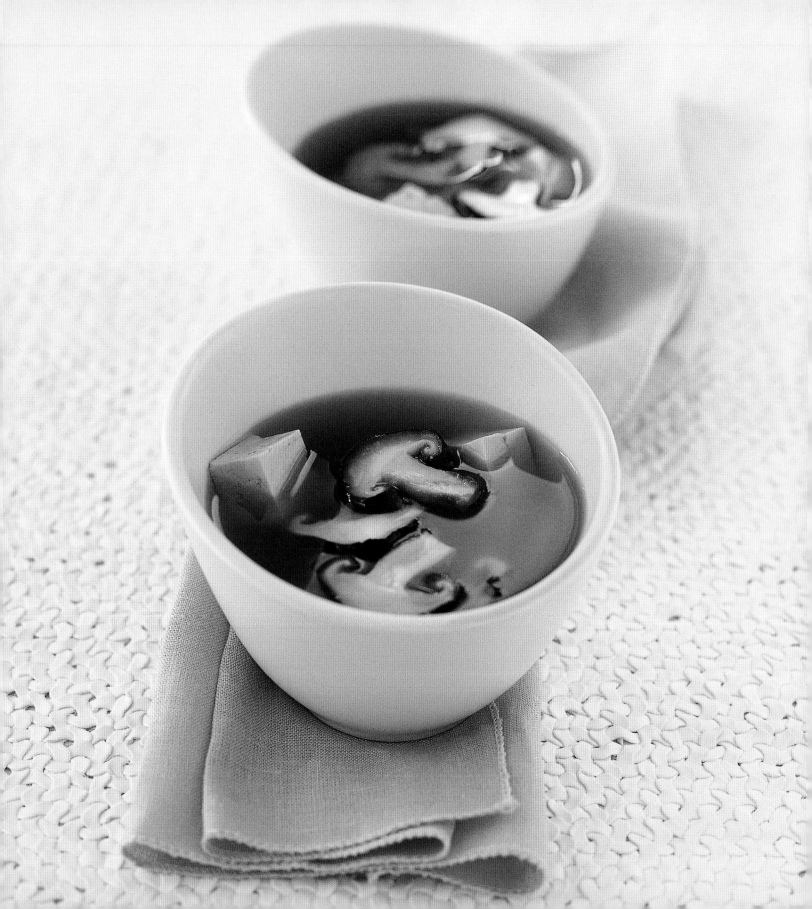

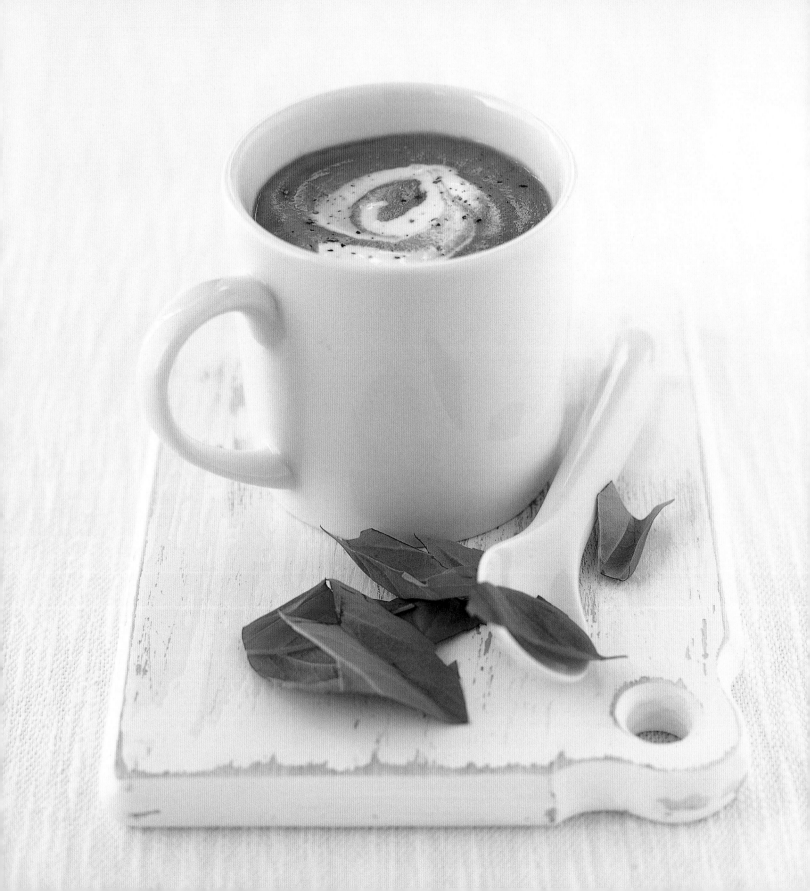

ROASTED PEPPER
AND TOMATO SOUP

serves 4

preparation time 10 minutes

cooking time 40 minutes

nutritional values per serving

Kcals 96 (396 kj) Protein 3 g Carb 16 g Fat 3 g

Saturated fat 1 g Fibre 5 g

---

4 red peppers, cored and deseeded

500 g (1 lb) tomatoes, halved

1 teaspoon olive oil

1 onion, chopped

1 carrot, chopped

600 ml (1 pint) Vegetable Stock (*see page 55*)

2 tablespoons light crème fraîche

handful of basil, torn

pepper

1 Place the peppers skin-side up and the tomatoes skin-side down on a baking sheet under a high grill and cook for 8–10 minutes until the skins of the peppers are blackened.

2 Remove the peppers and place them in a plastic bag. Fold over the top to seal and leave to cool, then remove the skins and slice the flesh. Leave the tomatoes to cool, then remove the skins.

3 Meanwhile, heat the oil in a large saucepan, add the onion and carrot and fry for 5 minutes. Add the stock and the skinned roasted peppers and tomatoes, bring to the boil and simmer for 25 minutes until the carrot is tender.

4 Transfer the soup to a liquidizer or food processor and blend until smooth. Return to the pan and heat through. Stir through the crème fraîche and basil, season well with pepper and serve.

SMOKY BACON
AND WHITE BEAN SOUP

serves 4

preparation time 5 minutes

cooking time 15 minutes

nutritional values per serving

Kcals 136 (562 kj) Protein 11 g Carb 21 g Fat 2 g

Saturated fat 0 g Fibre 10 g

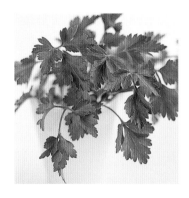

1 teaspoon olive oil

2 smoked bacon rashers, chopped

2 garlic cloves, crushed

1 onion, chopped

few thyme or lemon thyme sprigs

2 x 400 g (13 oz) cans cannellini beans, drained and rinsed

1 quantity Vegetable Stock (*see page 55*)

2 tablespoons chopped parsley

pepper

fresh bread, to serve

1 Heat the oil in a large saucepan, add the bacon, garlic and onion and fry for 3–4 minutes until the bacon is beginning to brown and the onion to soften.

2 Add the thyme and continue to fry for 1 minute. Then add the beans and stock to the pan, bring to the boil and simmer for 10 minutes.

3 Transfer the soup to a liquidizer or food processor and blend with the parsley and pepper until smooth. Return to the pan, heat through and serve with fresh bread.

POTATO, AVOCADO
AND SUN-BLUSH TOMATO SALAD

serves 4

preparation time 10 minutes, plus cooling

cooking time 15 minutes

nutritional values per serving

Kcals 312 (1310 kj) Protein 3 g Carb 35 g Fat 16 g

Saturated fat 4 g Fibre 3 g

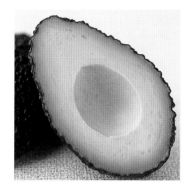

750 g (1½ lb) new potatoes

2 tablespoons fat-free French dressing

2 tablespoons light crème fraîche

1 large avocado, peeled, stoned and sliced

1 punnet of cress

75 g (3 oz) sun-blush or sun-dried tomatoes, sliced

1 bunch of spring onions, sliced

pepper

1 Place the potatoes in a saucepan of boiling water and cook for 12–15 minutes until tender. Drain, then tip into a bowl and cut up any of the potatoes that are too large to be bite-sized.

2 Add the dressing and crème fraîche to the potatoes, stir together, then leave to cool for 20 minutes.

3 Tip in the remaining ingredients and add plenty of pepper, mix well and serve.

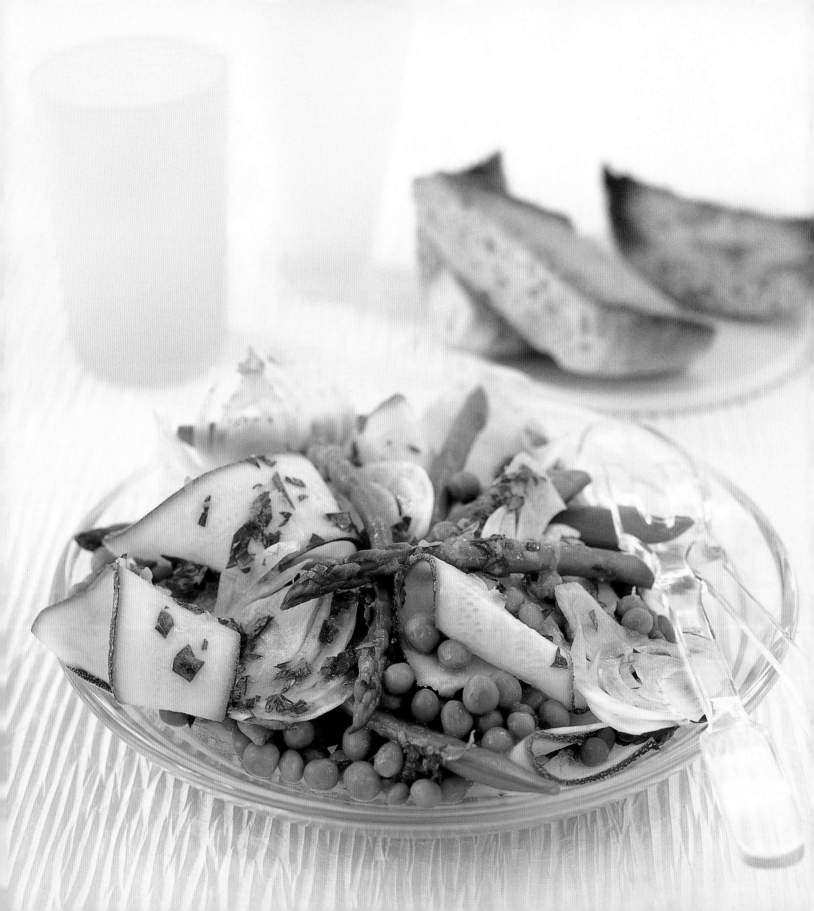

SPRING VEGETABLE SALAD
WITH HEALTHY GARLIC BREAD

serves 4

preparation time 10 minutes

cooking time 10 minutes

nutritional values per serving

Kcals 325 (1342 kj) Protein 17 g Carb 40 g Fat 11 g

Saturated fat 1 g Fibre 8 g

---

200 g (7 oz) fresh or frozen peas

200 g (7 oz) asparagus, trimmed

200 g (7 oz) sugar snap peas

**2 courgettes, cut into long thin ribbons
with a vegetable peeler**

1 fennel bulb, very thinly sliced

grated rind and juice of 1 lemon

1 teaspoon Dijon mustard

1 teaspoon clear honey

1 tablespoon chopped parsley

2 tablespoons olive oil

for the garlic bread

4 ciabatta rolls, halved

1 garlic clove

1 Place the peas, asparagus and sugar snap peas in a saucepan of boiling water and simmer for 3 minutes. Drain, then refresh under cold running water.

2 Place the vegetables in a large bowl with the courgette ribbons and fennel and mix together.

3 Whisk together the lemon rind and juice, mustard, honey, parsley and half the oil in a separate bowl. Toss this dressing through the vegetables.

4 Rub the cut sides of the rolls with the garlic clove, drizzle over the remaining oil, then place the rolls on a baking sheet under a high grill and toast on both sides. Serve with the salad.

LENTIL SALAD
WITH GREEN SALSA

serves 4

preparation time 15 minutes

cooking time 45 minutes

nutritional values per serving

Kcals 423 (1747 kj) Protein 22 g Carb 75 g Fat 6 g

Saturated fat 1 g Fibre 7 g

---

1 teaspoon olive oil

1 small onion, finely chopped

300 g (10 oz) Puy lentils

450 ml (¾ pint) Vegetable Stock (*see page 55*)

200 g (7 oz) cherry tomatoes, chopped

1 bunch of spring onions, shredded

4 chapatis or flat breads, toasted, to serve

for the salsa

4 tablespoons chopped mixed herbs, e.g., parsley, coriander and chives

1 tablespoon capers, drained

2 anchovy fillets (optional)

1 tablespoon olive oil

grated rind and juice of 1 lime

1 Heat the oil in a medium saucepan, add the onion and fry for 2–3 minutes until beginning to soften.

2 Add the lentils and stock, bring to the boil, then cover and simmer for 30–40 minutes until the lentils are tender and the stock has been absorbed. Add the tomatoes and spring onions and stir well.

3 Meanwhile, place the salsa ingredients in a liquidizer or food processor and blend for a few seconds until combined but still retaining a little texture.

4 Drizzle the salsa over the warm lentils and toss together. Serve with toasted chapatis or flat breads.

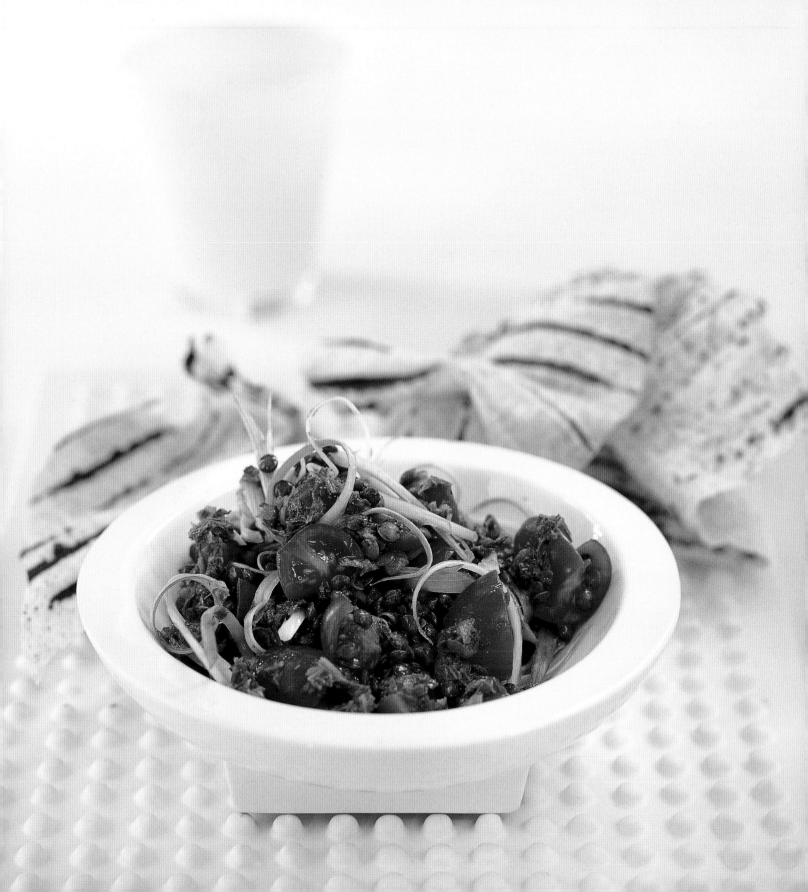

SMOKED MACKEREL SALAD
WITH ORANGE AND WATERCRESS

serves 4

preparation time 5 minutes, plus cooling and standing

cooking time 10 minutes

nutritional values per serving

Kcals 333 (1375 kj) Protein 13 g Carb 36 g Fat 15 g

Saturated fat 4 g Fibre 4 g

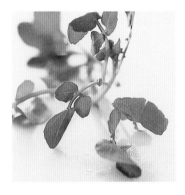

125 g (4 oz) long-grain rice

125 g (4 oz) wild rice

2 large peppered smoked mackerel fillets, skinned and flaked

3 oranges, segmented

1 large bunch of watercress, roughly torn

50 g (2 oz) mixed seeds, e.g. pumpkin and sunflower, toasted

75 g (3 oz) feta cheese, crumbled

granary bread, to serve

1 Cook the long-grain and wild rice, according to the packet instructions, then drain and leave to cool.

2 Mix together the remaining ingredients in a large bowl, then add the cooled rice.

3 Cover and set aside for about 10 minutes to allow the flavours to develop, then serve with granary bread.

CAMARGUE

RED RICE SALAD

serves 4
preparation time 10 minutes
cooking time 30 minutes

nutritional values per serving

Kcals 349 (1441 kj) Protein 7 g Carb 54 g Fat 13 g
Saturated fat 3 g Fibre 3 g

---

250 g (8 oz) Camargue red rice

1 bunch spring onions, sliced

2 tablespoons ready-made pesto

1 large avocado, peeled, stoned and sliced

200 g (7 oz) cherry tomatoes, chopped

75 g (3 oz) rocket

1 tablespoon balsamic vinegar

1 Cook the rice according to the packet instructions, then drain. Leave to cool.

2 Mix together the rice and the remaining ingredients in a large bowl.

3 Serve the salad on its own, or with meat or fish for a barbecue.

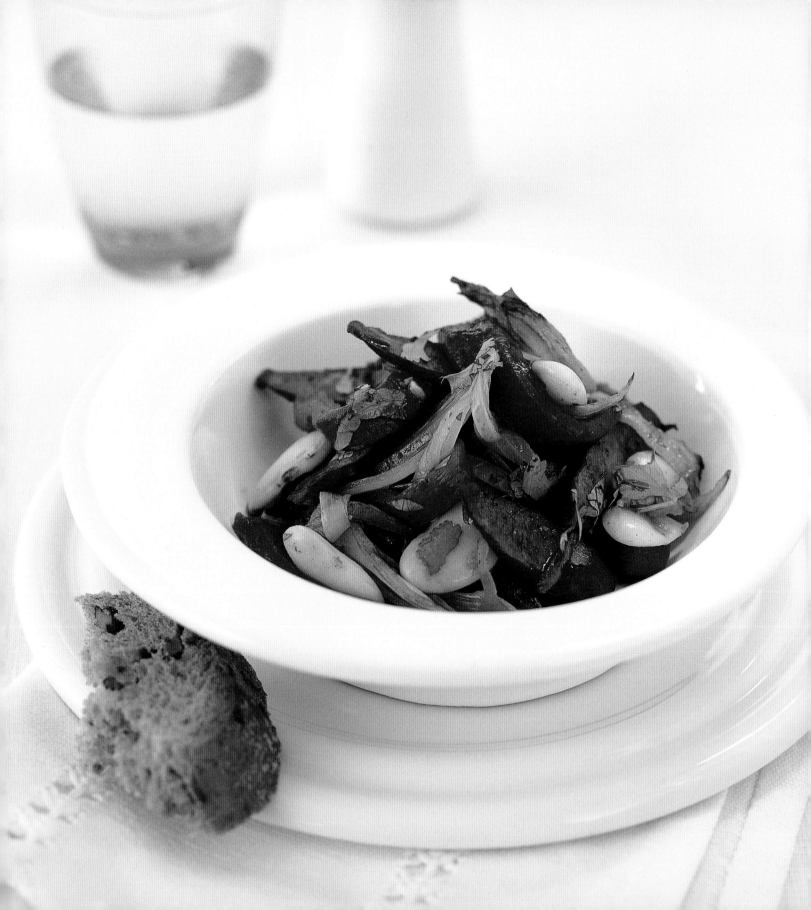

BEAN, KABANOS
AND ROASTED PEPPER SALAD

serves 4

preparation time 10 minutes

cooking time 20 minutes

nutritional values per serving

Kcals 270 (1115 kj) Protein 13 g Carb 27 g Fat 12 g

Saturated fat 1 g Fibre 10 g

---

3 red peppers, cored and deseeded

1 red chilli, deseeded

1 tablespoon olive oil

1 onion, sliced

75 g (3 oz) kabanos sausage, thinly sliced

2 x 400 g (13 oz) cans butter or flageolet beans, drained and rinsed

1 tablespoon balsamic vinegar

2 tablespoons chopped coriander

walnut bread, to serve

1 Place the peppers and chilli skin-side up on a baking sheet under a high grill and cook for 8–10 minutes until the skins are blackened.

2 Remove the peppers and chilli and place them in a plastic bag. Fold over the top to seal and leave to cool, then remove the skins and slice the flesh.

3 Meanwhile, heat the oil in a nonstick frying pan, add the onion and fry for 5–6 minutes until soft. Add the kabanos sausage and fry for 1–2 minutes until crisp.

4 Add all the remaining ingredients and mix well. Serve the salad with walnut bread.

TURKEY AND AVOCADO SALAD
WITH TOASTED SEEDS

serves 4

preparation time 10 minutes

cooking time no cooking

nutritional values per serving

Kcals 290 (1198 kj) Protein 29 g Carb 5 g Fat 17 g

Saturated fat 3 g Fibre 2 g

---

350 g (12 oz) cooked turkey, sliced

1 large avocado, peeled, stoned and sliced

1 punnet mustard and cress

150 g (5 oz) mixed salad leaves

50 g (2 oz) mixed seeds, e.g., pumpkin and sunflower, toasted

wholegrain rye bread, toasted or flat breads, to serve

for the dressing

2 tablespoons apple juice

2 tablespoons low-fat natural yogurt

1 teaspoon clear honey

1 teaspoon wholegrain mustard

1 Toss together all the salad ingredients in a large bowl.

2 Whisk together the dressing ingredients in a separate bowl. Pour over the salad and toss to coat.

3 Serve with toasted wholegrain rye bread or rolled up in flat breads.

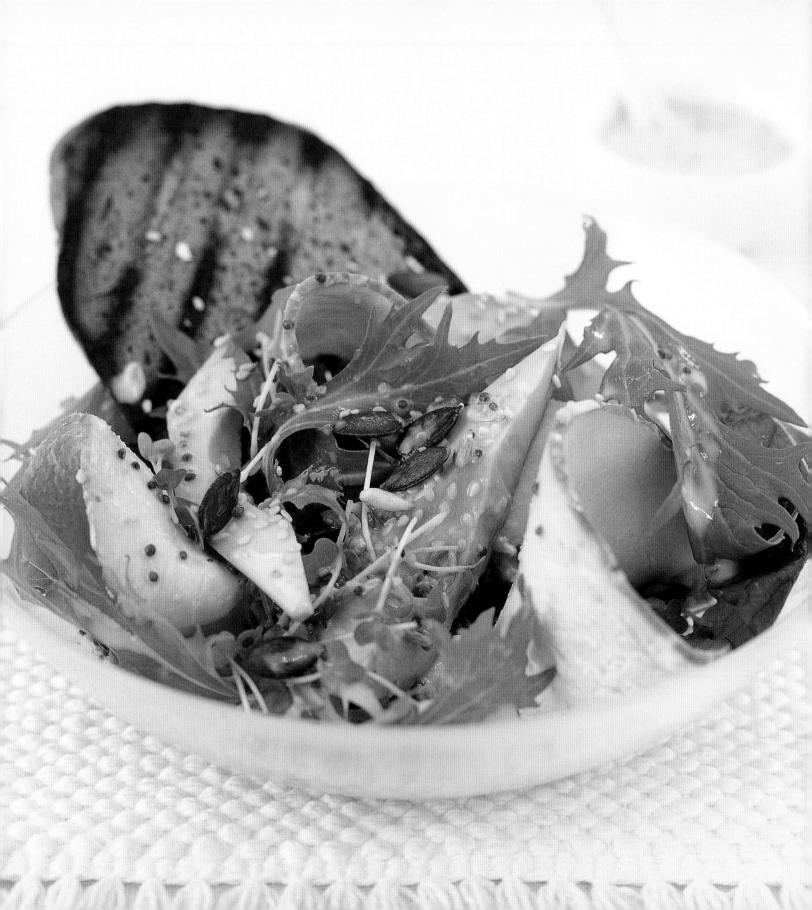

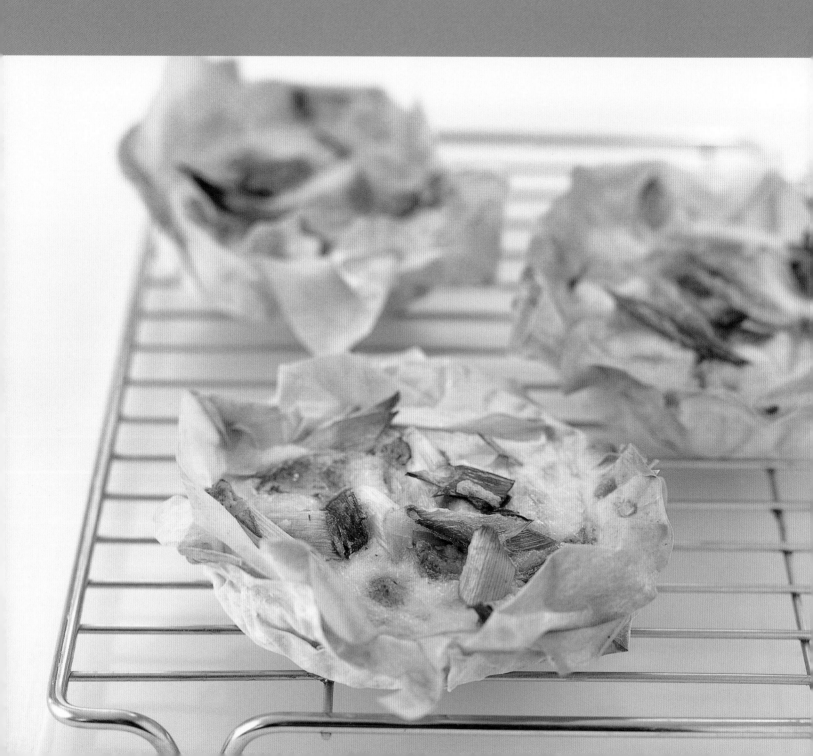

EASY ENTERTAINING

STILTON AND LEEK
TARTLETS

serves 4

preparation time 15 minutes

cooking time 25 minutes

nutritional values per serving

Kcals 148 (611 kj) Protein 8 g Carb 7 g Fat 10 g

Saturated fat 5 g Fibre 1 g

---

1 teaspoon olive oil

8 baby leeks, finely sliced

50 g (2 oz) Stilton cheese, crumbled

1 teaspoon chopped thyme

2 eggs, beaten

4 tablespoons light crème fraîche

12 x 15 cm (6 inch) squares filo pastry

milk, for brushing

mixed salad, to serve

1 Heat the oil in a saucepan, add the leeks and fry for 3–4 minutes until softened.

2 Stir half the Stilton and the thyme into the leek mixture, then blend together the remaining Stilton, the eggs and crème fraîche in a bowl.

3 Brush the filo squares with a little milk and use them to line 4 x 10-cm (4-inch) fluted flan tins. Divide the leek mixture between the tins, then pour over the cheese and egg mixture.

4 Place the tins on a baking sheet and bake in a preheated oven, 200°C (400°F), Gas Mark 6, for 15–20 minutes until the filling is set. Serve with a mixed salad.

CHICKEN LIVER PÂTÉ
WITH PEPPERCORNS

serves 4

preparation time 5 minutes, plus chilling

cooking time 30 minutes

nutritional values per serving

Kcals 151 (624 kj) Protein 12 g Carb 1 g Fat 11 g

Saturated fat 6 g Fibre 0 g

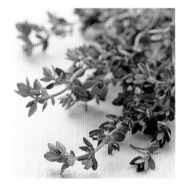

1 onion, cut into chunks

1 garlic clove

250 g (8 oz) chicken livers

25 g (1 oz) unsalted butter

2 thyme sprigs

4 tablespoons light crème fraîche

1 tablespoon green peppercorns in brine, drained

pepper

Olive and Haloumi Bread *(see page 152)*, **to serve**

1 Place the onion, garlic, chicken livers, butter and thyme in an ovenproof dish and cook in a preheated oven, 200°C (400°F), Gas Mark 6, for 25–30 minutes until the onions are tender.

2 Remove the dish from the oven, leave to cool a little, then transfer to a liquidizer or food processor with the crème fraîche. Blend until smooth and stir through the peppercorns.

3 Divide between 4 ramekins, cover and refrigerate for 2 hours. Serve with slices of olive and haloumi bread.

FRENCH ONION SOUP
WITH CHEESY TOPPERS

serves 4

preparation time 10 minutes

cooking time 35 minutes

nutritional values per serving

Kcals 226 (933 kj) Protein 8 g Carb 31 g Fat 6 g

Saturated fat 3 g Fibre 2 g

1 teaspoon olive oil

500 g (1 lb) large onions, thinly sliced

2 garlic cloves, crushed

pinch of sugar

1 thyme sprig

900 ml (1½ pints) beef stock (made with concentrated liquid stock)

125 ml (4 fl oz) dry white wine

pepper

for the cheesy toppers

8 slices French bread

50 g (2 oz) Gruyère cheese, grated

1 Heat the oil in a large saucepan, add the onions, garlic and sugar and cook over a medium heat for 10–12 minutes until softened and beginning to turn golden.

2 Add the thyme, stock and wine, bring to the boil and simmer for 20 minutes. Season well with pepper.

3 Toast the bread under a high grill on one side, then top the untoasted side with the cheese. Place it back under the grill and cook for 1–2 minutes until golden and bubbling.

4 Ladle the soup into bowls and serve with the cheesy toppers.

RED PEPPER AND FETA ROLLS
WITH OLIVES

serves 4

preparation time 10 minutes, plus cooling

cooking time 10 minutes

nutritional values per serving

Kcals 146 (603 kJ) Protein 6 g Carb 5 g Fat 11 g

Saturated fat 4 g Fibre 2 g

---

2 red peppers, cored, deseeded and quartered lengthways

100 g (3½ oz) feta cheese, thinly sliced or crumbled

16 basil leaves

16 black olives, pitted and halved

15 g (½ oz) pine nuts, toasted

1 tablespoon ready-made pesto

1 tablespoon ready-made fat-free French dressing

to serve

rocket

crusty bread

1 Place the peppers skin-side up on a baking sheet under a high grill and cook for 7–8 minutes until the skins are blackened.

2 Remove the peppers and place them in a plastic bag. Fold over the top to seal and leave to cool for 20 minutes, then remove the skins.

3 Lay the skinned pepper quarters on a board and layer up the feta, basil leaves, olives and pine nuts on each one.

4 Carefully roll up the peppers and secure with a cocktail stick. Place 2 pepper rolls on each serving plate.

5 Whisk together the pesto and French dressing in a small bowl and drizzle over the pepper rolls. Serve with rocket and some crusty bread to mop up the juices.

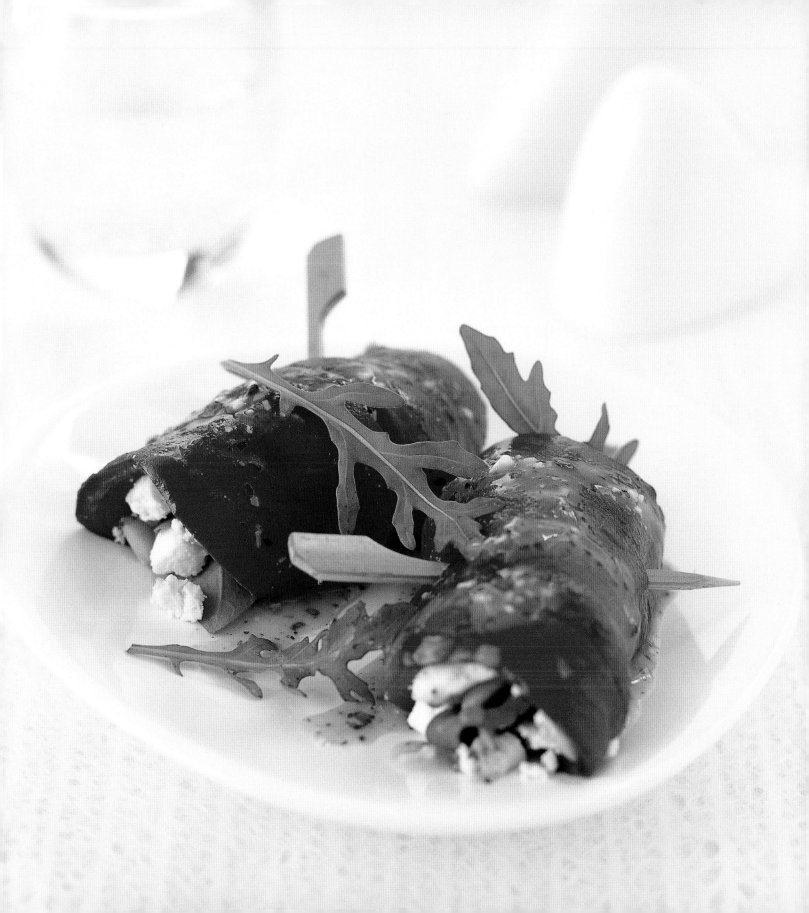

MARINATED PRAWNS
WITH MANGO

serves 4

preparation time 10 minutes, plus marinating

cooking time 5 minutes

nutritional values per serving

Kcals 115 (475 kj) Protein 11 g Carb 15 g Fat 1 g

Saturated fat 0 g Fibre 2 g

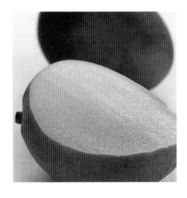

1 garlic clove

grated rind and juice of 1 lime

4 spring onions, roughly chopped

1 teaspoon clear honey

1 tablespoon chopped mint

1 tablespoon chopped coriander

24 raw peeled king prawns

1 teaspoon oil

2 mangoes, peeled, stoned and thinly sliced

toasted ciabatta, to serve

1 Place the garlic, lime rind and juice, spring onions, honey, mint and coriander in a liquidizer or food processor and blend for a few seconds until combined but still retaining a little texture.

2 Tip the mixture into a non-metallic bowl, then stir in the prawns, cover and leave to marinate in a cool place for a few minutes.

3 Heat the oil in a nonstick frying pan, add the prawns and marinade and fry for 2–3 minutes until the prawns have turned pink and are cooked through. Add the mango and mix well, then serve with slices of toasted ciabatta.

BEEF SKEWERS
WITH DIPPING SAUCE

serves 4

preparation time 10 minutes, plus marinating

cooking time 5 minutes

nutritional values per serving

Kcals 140 (578 kj) Protein 18 g Carb 2 g Fat 6 g

Saturated fat 2 g Fibre 0 g

---

1 tablespoon sweet chilli sauce

½ teaspoon cumin seeds, toasted

½ teaspoon ground coriander

1 teaspoon olive oil

350 g (12 oz) lean rump steak, cut into strips

for the sauce

1 tablespoon sweet chilli sauce

1 teaspoon Thai fish sauce

1 teaspoon white wine vinegar

to serve

2 tablespoons chopped coriander

1 tablespoon unsalted peanuts, roughly chopped (optional)

1 Mix together the sweet chilli sauce, cumin seeds, ground coriander and oil in a non-metallic bowl. Add the meat and stir well to coat, then cover and leave to marinate in a cool place for 30 minutes.

2 Thread the meat on to 4 bamboo skewers that have been soaked in water for at least 20 minutes. Cook on a hot griddle or under a high grill for 2–3 minutes until cooked through.

3 Meanwhile, mix together the sauce ingredients in a small serving bowl. Serve the skewers with the sauce, scattered with the coriander and peanuts, if desired.

LEMON GRASS

FISH SKEWERS

serves 4
preparation time 5 minutes
cooking time 5 minutes

nutritional values per serving
Kcals 106 (438 kj) Protein 19 g Carb 0 g Fat 3 g
Saturated fat 0 g Fibre 0 g

---

500 g (1 lb) skinless haddock fillets, chopped

1 tablespoon chopped mint

2 tablespoons coriander

2 teaspoons red Thai curry paste

2 lime leaves, finely chopped, or the grated rind of 1 lime

2 lemon grass stalks, quartered lengthways

oil, for brushing

to serve

sweet chilli sauce

lime wedges

1 Place the fish, mint, coriander, curry paste and lime leaves or rind in a liquidizer or food processor and blend for 30 seconds until well combined.

2 Divide the mixture into 8 portions, then form each around a lemon grass stalk 'skewer'.

3 Brush with a little oil, then place under a high grill and cook for 4–5 minutes until cooked through. Serve with a little sweet chilli sauce and lime wedges.

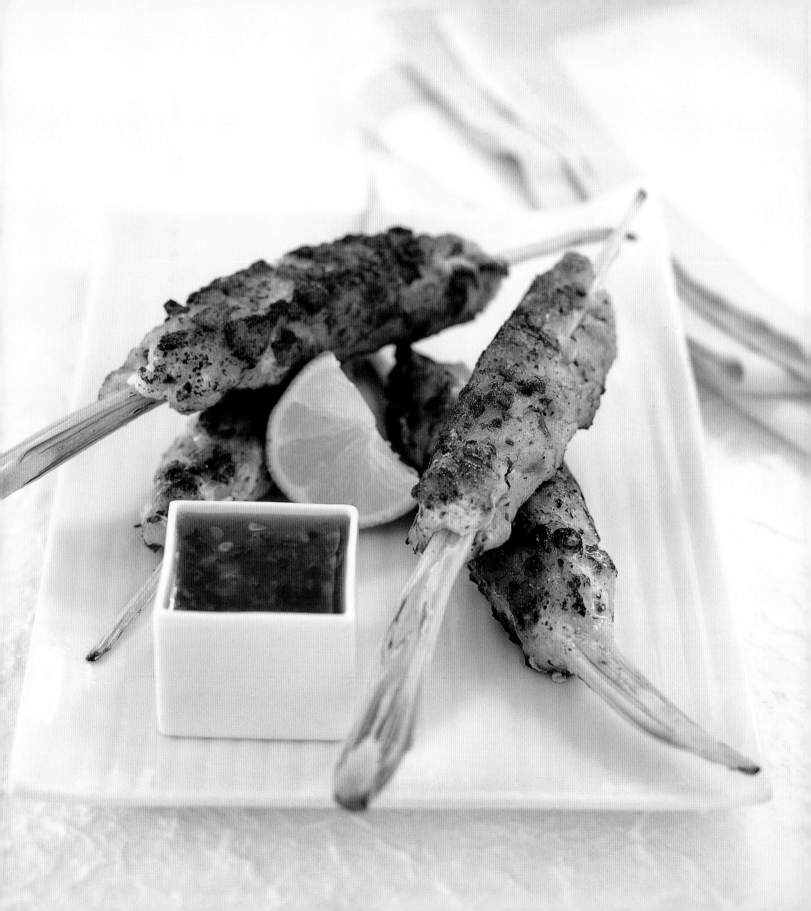

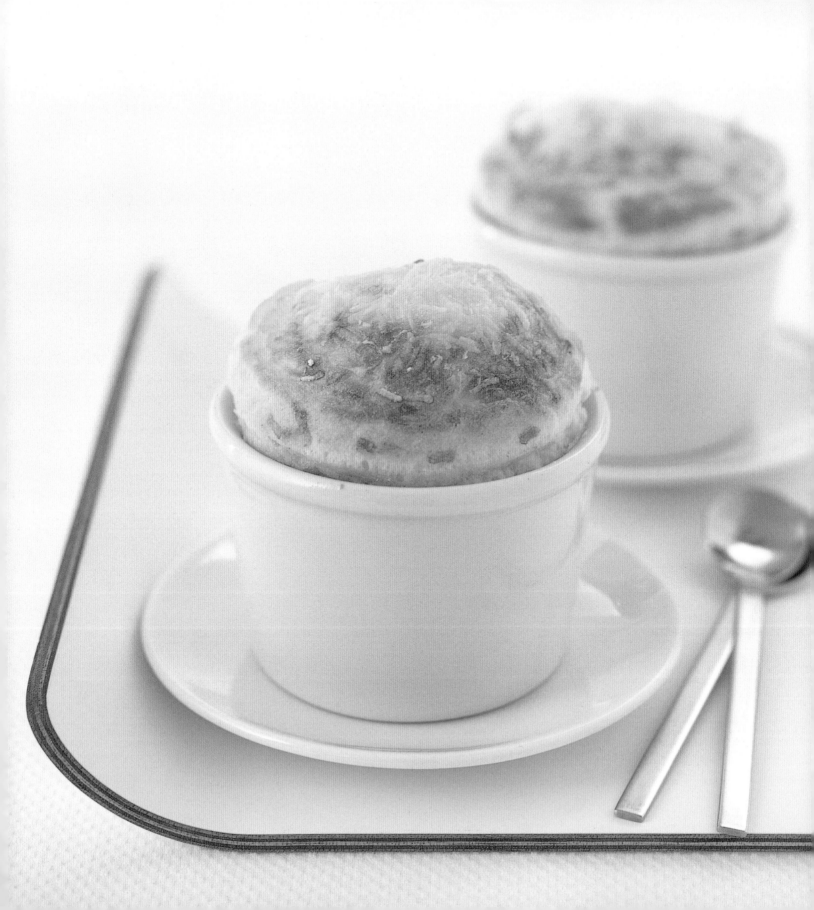

GOATS' CHEESE
AND HERB SOUFFLÉS

serves 4

preparation time 10 minutes

cooking time 15 minutes

nutritional values per serving

Kcals 277 (1144 kj) Protein 15 g Carb 13 g Fat 18 g

Saturated fat 7 g Fibre 1 g

---

25 g (1 oz) polyunsaturated margarine

50 g (2 oz) plain flour

300 ml (½ pint) semi-skimmed milk

4 eggs, separated

100 g (3½ oz) goats' cheese, crumbled

1 tablespoon chopped mixed herbs, e.g.,
parsley, chives and thyme

1 tablespoon freshly grated Parmesan cheese

salt and pepper

to serve

75 g (3 oz) rocket

2 tablespoons fat-free salad dressing

1 Melt the margarine in a medium saucepan, add the flour and cook, stirring, for 1 minute. Gradually add the milk, whisking all the time, and cook for 2 minutes until thickened.

2 Remove the pan from the heat. Beat in the egg yolks one at a time, then stir in the goats' cheese. Season well.

3 Whisk the eggs whites in a large bowl until they form firm peaks, then gradually fold them into the cheese mixture with the herbs. Transfer to 4 lightly oiled ramekins, sprinkle over the Parmesan, then bake in a preheated oven, 190°C (375°F), Gas Mark 5, for 10–12 minutes until risen and golden.

4 Toss together the rocket and dressing and serve with the soufflés.

THAI CHICKEN SHELLS
WITH CORIANDER AND COCONUT RICE

serves 4

preparation time 10 minutes

cooking time 15 minutes

nutritional values per serving

Kcals 276 (1139 kj) Protein 18 g Carb 33 g Fat 6 g

Saturated fat 1 g Fibre 0 g

1 teaspoon oil

2 large chicken breasts, about 150 g (4 oz) each, sliced

1 tablespoon red or green Thai curry paste

400 ml (14 fl oz) can coconut milk

for the rice

250 g (8 oz) basmati rice

100 ml (3½ fl oz) water

3 tablespoons chopped coriander

to serve

3 spring onions, sliced

4 Little Gem lettuces, separated into individual leaves

2 limes, cut into wedges

1 Heat the oil in a nonstick frying pan, add the chicken and fry for 2 minutes.

2 Add the curry paste and continue to fry for 1 minute, then add half the coconut milk, bring to the boil and simmer gently for 10 minutes.

3 Meanwhile, place the rice in a saucepan with the remaining coconut milk and measurement water. Bring to the boil, then cover and simmer for 10–12 minutes until the liquid is absorbed, adding a little extra water if necessary. Stir through the coriander.

4 To serve, place a little chicken, spring onion and rice on to a lettuce leaf and squeeze the lime wedges over the filled shells before eating.

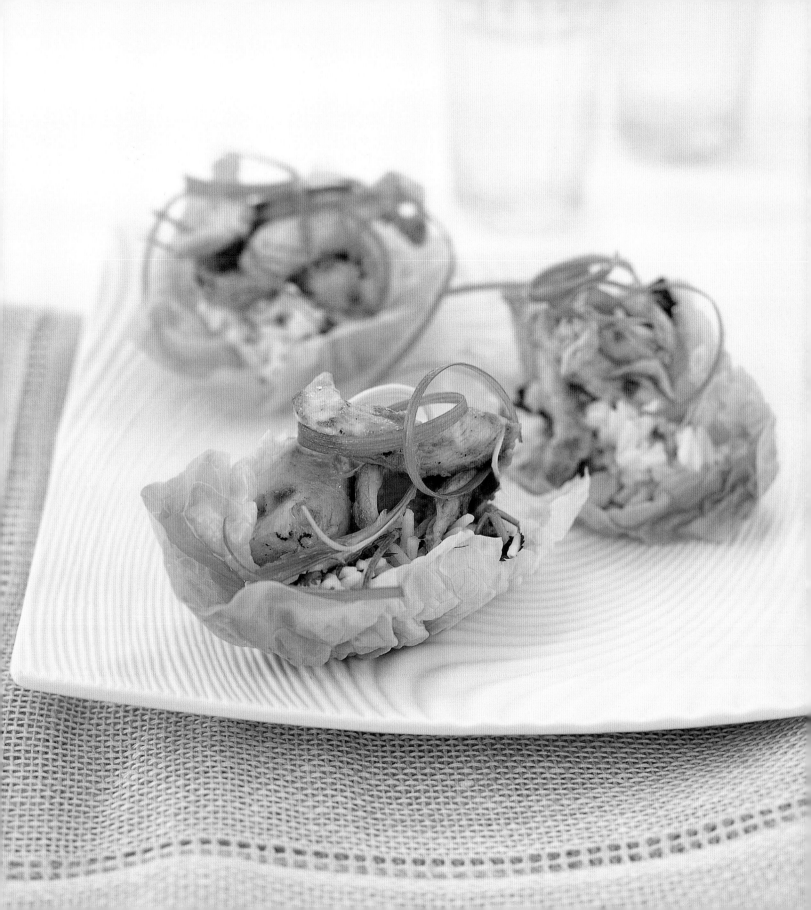

ONE-POT CHICKEN
STUFFED WITH SPRING HERBS

serves 4

preparation time 10 minutes

cooking time 45 minutes

nutritional values per serving

Kcals 275 (1135 kj) Protein 31 g Carb 22 g Fat 7 g

Saturated fat 3 g Fibre 3 g

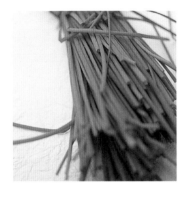

500 g (1 lb) new potatoes

4 boneless, skinless chicken breasts, about 125 g (4 oz) each

6 tablespoons mixed herbs, e.g., parsley, chives, chervil and mint

1 garlic clove, crushed

6 tablespoons light crème fraîche

8 baby leeks

2 heads chicory, halved lengthways

150 ml (¼ pint) chicken stock (made with concentrated liquid stock)

pepper

1 Place the potatoes in a saucepan of boiling water and cook for 12–15 minutes until tender. Drain, then cut into bite-sized pieces.

2 Make a slit lengthways down the side of each chicken breast to form a pocket, ensuring that you don't cut all the way through. Mix together the herbs, garlic and crème fraiche, season well with pepper, then spoon a little into each chicken pocket.

3 Place the leeks, chicory and potatoes in an ovenproof dish. Pour over the stock, then lay the chicken breasts on top. Spoon over the remaining herb mixture, then bake in a preheated oven, 200°C (400°F), Gas Mark 6, for 25–30 minutes. This one-pot dish needs no side dishes to accompany it.

STUFFED PORK TENDERLOIN
WITH APRICOTS AND WALNUTS

serves 4

preparation time 10 minutes

cooking time 20 minutes

nutritional values per serving

Kcals 404 (1689 kj) Protein 32 g Carb 13 g Fat 22 g

Saturated fat 7 g Fibre 3 g

---

500 g (1 lb) pork tenderloin

12 sage leaves, chopped

125 g (4 oz) ready-to-eat dried apricots, chopped

50 g (2 oz) walnuts, toasted and roughly chopped

50 g (2 oz) crumbly hard cheese, e.g., Wensleydale or Cheshire, crumbled

2 teaspoons olive oil

150 ml (¼ pint) chicken stock (made with concentrated liquid stock)

4 tablespoons light crème fraîche

to serve

seasonal vegetables

couscous or rice

1 Make a slit lengthways down the piece of pork and open it out. Lay the pork over a piece of clingfilm or baking parchment and gently flatten it with a rolling pin.

2 Mix together the sage, apricots, walnuts and cheese and spread the mixture over the pork, leaving a 1-cm (½-inch) gap all round the edge. Roll up and secure with cocktail sticks.

3 Heat the oil in a large, nonstick frying pan, add the rolled-up pork and fry for 3–4 minutes, turning to brown all over. Pour over the stock, then cover and simmer for 10–12 minutes until the pork is cooked through and the cheesy stuffing is beginning to ooze.

4 Remove the pork from the pan and slice on to warmed serving plates. Add the crème fraîche to the juices in the pan and heat through gently before pouring over the pork. Serve with seasonal vegetables and couscous or rice.

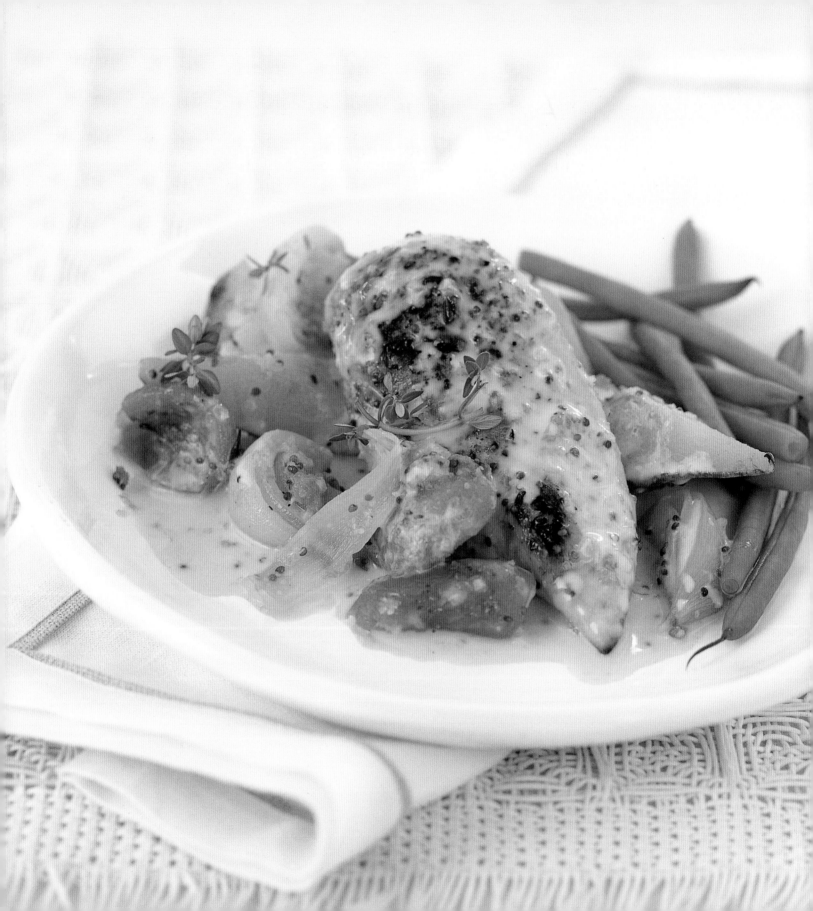

SWEET-GLAZED CHICKEN
WITH BAKED PEARS AND APRICOTS

serves 4

preparation time 10 minutes

cooking time 45 minutes

nutritional values per serving

Kcals 324 (1338 kj) Protein 30 g Carb 36 g Fat 7 g

Saturated fat 3 g Fibre 5 g

---

2 teaspoons olive oil

4 boneless, skinless chicken breasts, about 150 g (5 oz) each

8 fresh apricots, halved and stoned

2 pears, peeled, quartered and cored

500 g (1 lb) new potatoes

1 onion, cut into wedges

grated rind and juice of 2 oranges

few thyme sprigs, chopped

1 tablespoon wholegrain mustard

1 tablespoon clear honey

4 tablespoons light crème fraîche

pepper

to serve

green beans

sautéed spinach (optional)

1 Heat the oil in a nonstick frying pan, season the chicken with pepper and add to the pan. Fry for 2–3 minutes on each side until golden, then place in an ovenproof dish with the apricots, pears, potatoes and onion.

2 Mix together the orange rind and juice, thyme, mustard and honey and pour over the chicken. Cover the dish with foil and bake in a preheated oven, 180°C (350°F), Gas Mark 4, for 40 minutes, removing the foil halfway through cooking time.

3 When the chicken is cooked, stir the crème fraîche into the sauce before serving with green beans and sautéed spinach, if desired.

SESAME-CRUSTED SALMON
WITH STIR-FRIED VEGETABLES

serves 4

preparation time 10 minutes

cooking time 10 minutes

nutritional values per serving

Kcals 324 (1338 kj) Protein 23 g Carb 10 g Fat 20 g

Saturated fat 3 g Fibre 4 g

---

4 tablespoons sesame seeds

1 teaspoon dried chilli flakes

4 skinless salmon fillets, about 100 g (3½ oz) each

2 teaspoons olive oil

2 carrots, cut into matchsticks

2 red peppers, cored, deseeded and thinly sliced

200 g (7 oz) shiitake mushrooms, halved

2 pak choi, quartered lengthways

4 spring onions, shredded

1 tablespoon soy sauce

basmati rice, to serve

1 Mix together the sesame seeds and chilli flakes on a plate, then press the salmon pieces into this mixture to cover.

2 Heat half the oil in a nonstick frying pan or wok, add the salmon and cook over a medium heat for 3–4 minutes on each side until cooked through. Set the salmon aside, keeping it warm.

3 Heat the remaining oil in the pan, then add the vegetables and quickly stir-fry for 3–4 minutes until just cooked. Drizzle the soy sauce over the vegetables, then serve with the salmon and basmati rice.

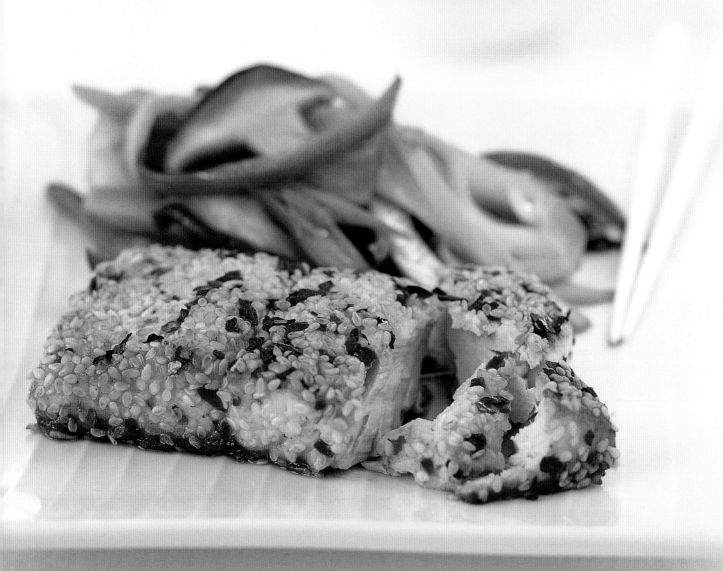

COD WITH OLIVE TAPENADE
AND SLICED POTATOES

serves 4

preparation time 15 minutes

cooking time 1 hour

nutritional values per serving

Kcals 322 (1329 kj) Protein 31 g Carb 38 g Fat 6 g

Saturated fat 1 g Fibre 4 g

---

for the potatoes

1 tablespoon olive oil

1 kg (2 lb) potatoes, thinly sliced

2 garlic cloves, thinly sliced

2 thyme sprigs, chopped

150 ml (¼ pint) Vegetable Stock (*see page 55*)

pepper

for the cod

4 thick cod loin fillets, about 150 g (5 oz) each

4 tablespoons dry white wine or stock

75 g (3 oz) black olives, pitted

1 anchovy fillet

2 tablespoons capers, drained

1 tablespoon chopped parsley

1 garlic clove

green salad, to serve

1 Lightly oil an ovenproof dish using 1 teaspoon of the oil. Layer up the potatoes, garlic and thyme, then mix together the stock and remaining oil and pour over the potatoes. Cover with foil and bake in a preheated oven, 160°C (325°F), Gas Mark 3, for 45 minutes, until tender.

2 Meanwhile, place the cod fillets in an ovenproof dish with the wine or stock. Place the olives, anchovy, capers, parsley and garlic in a liquidizer or food processor and blend together, then spoon this mixture on to the cod fillets.

3 Remove the foil from the potatoes and increase the oven temperature to 200°C (400°F), Gas Mark 6 to brown the top. Add the fish to the oven and cook for 15 minutes. Serve the fish and potatoes with a green salad.

SEAFOOD PIE
WITH CRUNCHY POTATO TOPPING

serves 4

preparation time 15 minutes

cooking time 40 minutes

nutritional values per serving

Kcals 433 (1788 kj) Protein 43 g Carb 46 g Fat 20 g

Saturated fat 8 g Fibre 3 g

---

25 g (1 oz) unsalted butter

1 onion, chopped

1 celery stick, diced

1 bay leaf

25 g (1 oz) plain flour

450 ml (¾ pint) semi-skimmed milk

500 g (1 lb) mixed skinless fish fillets, e.g., salmon and cod

250 g (8 oz) raw peeled prawns or king prawns

2 tablespoons chopped parsley

750 g (1½ lb) potatoes, cut into matchsticks

40 g (1½ oz) mature Cheddar cheese, grated

3 tablespoons light crème fraîche

pepper

to serve

steamed peas

steamed carrots

1 Melt the butter in a large saucepan, add the onion, celery and bay leaf and fry for 2–3 minutes until the onion begins to soften. Add the flour and cook, stirring, for 1 minute. Gradually add the milk, whisking all the time, and cook for 2 minutes until thickened. Season well with pepper.

2 Stir the fish, prawns and parsley into the sauce and simmer for 2 minutes, then transfer to an ovenproof dish.

3 Place the potato sticks in a saucepan of boiling water for 1 minute, then drain and mix with the Cheddar. Sprinkle over the fish. Dot the crème fraîche over the top, then bake in a preheated oven, 200°C (400°F), Gas Mark 6, for 25–30 minutes until golden and bubbling. Serve with steamed peas and carrots.

CHICKEN CURRY
WITH BABY SPINACH

serves 4

preparation time 10 minutes

cooking time 25 minutes

nutritional values per serving

Kcals 205 (847 kj) Protein 27 g Carb 10 g Fat 6 g

Saturated fat 2 g Fibre 2 g

---

1 tablespoon vegetable oil

4 boneless, skinless chicken breasts, about 125 g (4 oz) each, halved lengthways

1 onion, sliced

2 garlic cloves, chopped

1 green chilli, chopped

4 cardamom pods, lightly crushed

1 teaspoon cumin seeds

1 teaspoon dried chilli flakes

1 teaspoon ground ginger

1 teaspoon turmeric

250 g (8 oz) baby spinach leaves

300 g (10 oz) tomatoes, chopped

150 ml (¼ pint) light Greek yogurt

2 tablespoons chopped coriander

basmati rice, to serve

1 Heat the oil in a large nonstick saucepan or frying pan. Add the chicken, onion, garlic and chilli and fry for 4–5 minutes until the chicken begins to brown and the onion to soften.

2 Add the cardamom pods, cumin seeds, chilli flakes, ginger and turmeric and continue to fry for 1 minute.

3 Add the spinach to the pan, cover and cook gently until the spinach wilts, then stir in the tomatoes and simmer for 15 minutes, removing the lid for the last 5 minutes.

4 Stir in the yogurt and coriander and serve with basmati rice.

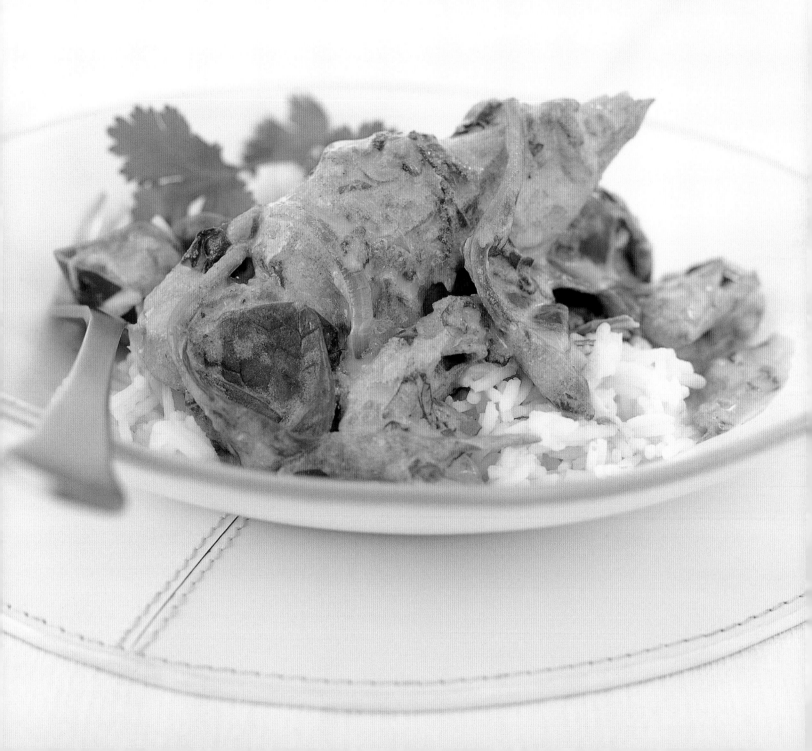

LAMB, FLAGEOLET BEAN
AND TOMATO WARMING POT

serves 4

preparation time 5 minutes

cooking time 1 hour 20 minutes

nutritional values per serving

Kcals 288 (1189 kj) Protein 27 g Carb 24 g Fat 9 g

Saturated fat 4 g Fibre 9 g

---

1 teaspoon olive oil

350 g (12 oz) lean lamb, cubed

16 pickling onions, peeled

1 garlic clove, crushed

1 tablespoon plain flour

600 ml (1 pint) lamb stock (made with concentrated liquid stock)

200 g (7 oz) can chopped tomatoes

1 bouquet garni

2 x 400 g (13 oz) cans flageolet beans, drained and rinsed

250 g (8 oz) cherry tomatoes

pepper

to serve

steamed potatoes

steamed green beans

1 Heat the oil in a flameproof casserole or saucepan, add the lamb and fry for 3–4 minutes until browned all over. Remove from the casserole and set aside.

2 Add the onions and garlic to the pan and fry for 4–5 minutes until the onions are beginning to brown.

3 Return the lamb and any juices to the pan, then stir through the flour and add the stock, canned tomatoes, bouquet garni and beans. Bring to the boil, stirring, then cover and simmer for 1 hour until the lamb is just tender.

4 Add the cherry tomatoes to the dish and season well with pepper Continue to simmer for 10 minutes then serve with steamed potatoes and green beans.

PASTA SHELLS
WITH RICH RABBIT SAUCE

serves 4

preparation time 10 minutes

cooking time 2 hours 10 minutes

nutritional values per serving

Kcals 515 (2127 kj) Protein 33 g Carb 71 g Fat 7 g

Saturated fat 2 g Fibre 3 g

---

1 teaspoon olive oil

1 onion, chopped

1 carrot, finely chopped

1 celery stick, diced

1 rabbit, jointed, or 4 chicken joints

1 teaspoon five-spice powder

1 tablespoon plain flour

pared rind of 1 orange

1 rosemary sprig

1 teaspoon chopped marjoram

300 ml (½ pint) red wine

300 ml (½ pint) beef stock (made with concentrated liquid stock)

350 g (12 oz) pasta shells

4 tablespoons light crème fraîche

pepper

green salad, to serve

1 Heat the oil in a large saucepan, add the onion, carrot and celery and fry for 2–3 minutes until softened. Add the rabbit or chicken and fry for 2–3 minutes until browned all over, then add the spice and flour and stir to combine.

2 Add the orange rind, rosemary and marjoram, then gradually stir in the wine and stock. Bring the mixture to the boil, then cover and simmer for about 2 hours until the rabbit or chicken is very tender. Carefully remove all the bones.

3 Meanwhile, cook the pasta according to the packet instructions, then drain. Add the rabbit or chicken, sauce and crème fraîche to the pasta and stir to combine. Serve with a green salad.

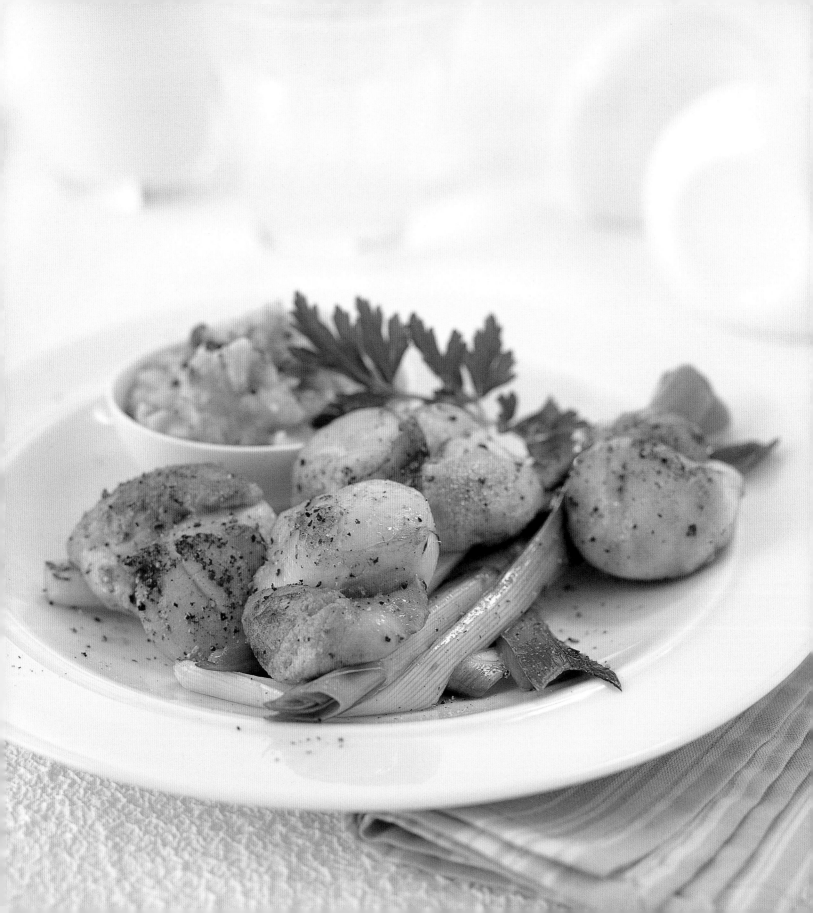

PAN-FRIED SCALLOPS
WITH WHITE BEAN PURÉE AND LEEKS

serves 4

preparation time 10 minutes

cooking time 15 minutes

nutritional values per serving

Kcals 293 (1210 kj) Protein 37 g Carb 27 g Fat 4 g

Saturated fat 1 g Fibre 9 g

---

2 x 400 g (13 oz) can cannellini beans, drained and rinsed

2 garlic cloves

200 ml (7 fl oz) Vegetable Stock (*see page 55*)

2 tablespoons chopped parsley

2 teaspoons olive oil

16 baby leeks

3 tablespoons water

16 large scallops, shelled and prepared

1 Place the beans, garlic and stock in a saucepan, bring to the boil and simmer for 10 minutes. Remove from the heat, drain off any excess liquid, then mash with a potato masher and stir in the parsley. Keep warm.

2 Heat half the oil in a nonstick frying pan, add the leeks and fry for 2 minutes, then add the measurement water. Cover and simmer for 5–6 minutes until tender.

3 Meanwhile, heat the remaining oil in a small frying pan, add the scallops and fry for 1 minute on each side. Serve with the white bean purée and leeks.

CLAM TAGLIATELLE

WITH RAGU SAUCE

serves 4

preparation time 5 minutes

cooking time 15 minutes

nutritional values per serving

Kcals 405 (1673 kj) Protein 24 g Carb 69 g Fat 3 g

Saturated fat 1 g Fibre 4 g

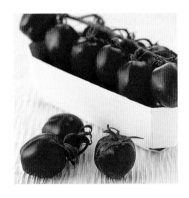

350 g (12 oz) tagliatelle

1 teaspoon oil

1 small onion, finely chopped

1 garlic clove, crushed

1 red chilli, finely chopped

1 kg (2 lb) clams in their shells, prepared

125 ml (4 fl oz) dry white wine

500 g (1 lb) cherry tomatoes, halved

handful of basil, torn

1 Cook the pasta according to the packet instructions, then drain and return to the pan to keep warm.

2 Meanwhile, heat the oil in a large saucepan, add the onion, garlic and chilli and fry for 2 minutes.

3 Add the clams, wine and tomatoes, then cover and cook for 3–5 minutes until all the clams are opened, discarding any that remain closed.

4 Add the pasta and basil and stir well to combine, then serve.

PAN-FRIED TIGER PRAWNS
WITH PANCETTA AND WATERCRESS

serves 4

preparation time 5 minutes

cooking time 10 minutes

nutritional values per serving

Kcals 187 (772 kj) Protein 28 g Carb 3 g Fat 6 g

Saturated fat 3 g Fibre 0 g

---

1 teaspoon olive oil

15 g (½ oz) unsalted butter

50 g (2 oz) pancetta or smoked bacon, finely chopped

500 g (1 lb) raw peeled tiger prawns

grated rind and juice of 1 lemon

1 large bunch of watercress

to serve

potatoes or pasta (unless served as an appetizer)

1 Heat the oil and butter in a large frying pan, add the pancetta or smoked bacon and fry for 3–4 minutes until crisp.

2 Add the prawns and fry for 1 minute on each side. Sprinkle over the lemon rind and juice and continue to fry for 1 minute, then add the watercress and combine well.

3 Serve as an appetizer or with potatoes or pasta as a main course.

LAMB CUTLETS
WITH HERBED CRUST AND GARLIC GREENS

serves 4

preparation time 10 minutes

cooking time 15 minutes

nutritional values per serving

Kcals 280 (1156 kj) Protein 25 g Carb 10 g Fat 15 g

Saturated fat 6 g Fibre 4 g

---

12 lean lamb cutlets, about 40 g (1½ oz) each

2 tablespoons ready-made pesto

3 tablespoons granary breadcrumbs

1 tablespoon chopped walnuts, toasted

for the garlic greens

1 teaspoon oil

2 garlic cloves, crushed

625 g (1¼ lb) greens, finely shredded and blanched

to serve

baby carrots

cabbage

1 Heat a nonstick frying pan or griddle until hot, add the cutlets and cook for 1 minute on each side, then transfer to a baking sheet.

2 Mix together the pesto, breadcrumbs and walnuts and use to top one side of the cutlets, pressing down lightly. Cook in a preheated oven, 200°C (400°F), Gas Mark 6, for 10–12 minutes.

3 Meanwhile, heat the oil in a frying pan or wok, add the garlic and stir-fry for 1 minute, then add the greens and continue to stir-fry for 3–4 minutes until tender.

4 Serve with the lamb along with baby carrots and cabbage.

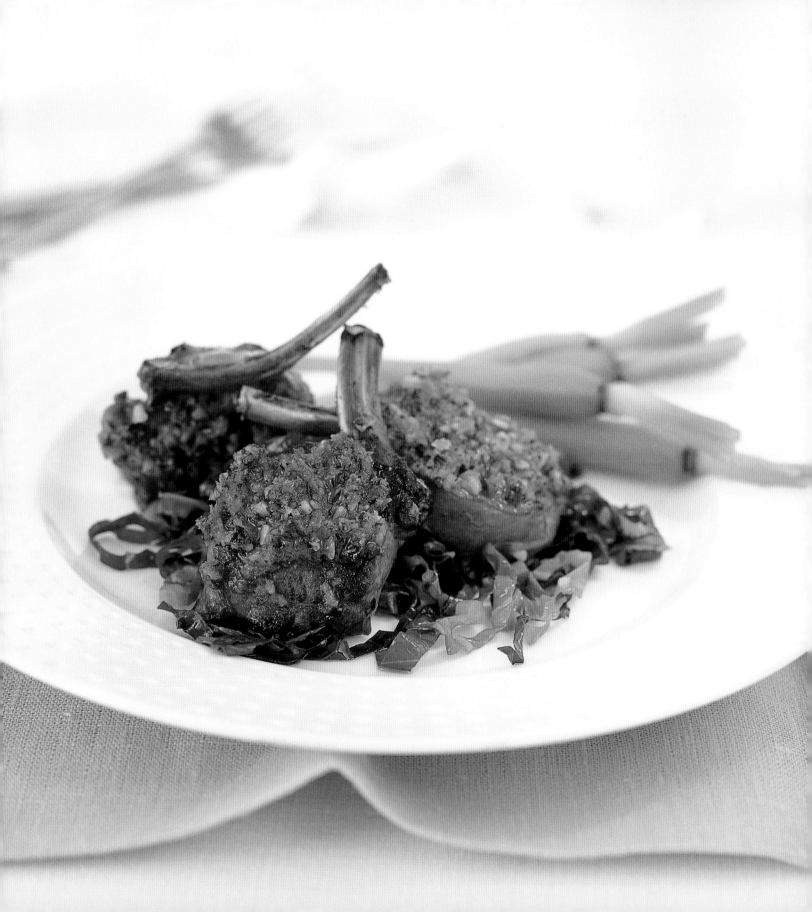

THAI NOODLE SALAD

WITH PRAWNS

serves 4

preparation time 10 minutes

cooking time 5 minutes

nutritional values per serving

Kcals 269 (1111 kj) Protein 23 g Carb 37 g Fat 4 g

Saturated fat 0 g Fibre 2 g

---

300 g (10 oz) rice noodles

2 carrots, peeled into long thin strips

½ cucumber, halved lengthways and thinly sliced

6 spring onions, shredded

125 g (4 oz) bean sprouts

handful of basil

500 g (1 lb) cooked peeled king prawns (or small prawns, if you prefer)

for the dressing

1 tablespoon sesame oil

2 tablespoons sesame seeds, toasted

2 red chillies, finely sliced

6 tablespoons chopped coriander

1 teaspoon Thai fish sauce

2 teaspoons caster sugar

1 Cook the rice noodles according to the packet instructions. Drain, then refresh under cold running water.

2 Place all the salad ingredients in a large bowl, including the noodles. Whisk together the dressing ingredients in a separate bowl, then drizzle this over the salad and toss well to combine before serving.

PAN-FRIED PLAICE
WITH CREAMY MUSTARD SAUCE

serves 4

preparation time 10 minutes

cooking time 10 minutes

nutritional values per serving

Kcals 182 (752 kj) Protein 27 g Carb 1 g Fat 5 g

Saturated fat 3 g Fibre 0 g

---

1 teaspoon olive oil

1 small onion, finely chopped

1 garlic clove, crushed

4 plaice or sole fillets, about 150 g (5 oz) each

125 ml (4 fl oz) dry white wine

2 tablespoons wholegrain mustard

200 g (7 oz) light crème fraîche

2 tablespoons chopped mixed herbs

to serve

rice or new potatoes

steamed vegetables

1 Heat the oil in a large frying pan, add the onion and garlic and fry for 3 minutes until softened.

2 Add the fish fillets and cook for 1 minute on each side. Then add the wine and simmer to reduce by half.

3 Stir through the remaining ingredients, bring to the boil and simmer for 3–4 minutes until the sauce has thickened slightly and the fish is tender.

4 Serve with rice or new potatoes and steamed vegetables.

ASPARAGUS AND DOLCELATTE
RISOTTO

serves 4

preparation time 10 minutes

cooking time 25 minutes

nutritional values per serving

Kcals 411 (1697 kj) Protein 11 g Carb 78 g Fat 8 g

Saturated fat 4 g Fibre 2 g

---

1 teaspoon olive oil

1 small onion, finely chopped

300 g (10 oz) asparagus, halved and the stem end finely sliced

350 g (12 oz) arborio rice

2 tablespoons dry white wine

1.2 litres (2 pints) Vegetable Stock (*see page 55*)

75 g (3 oz) dolcelatte cheese, chopped

2 tablespoons chopped parsley

rocket and tomato salad, to serve

1 Heat the oil in a large nonstick frying pan, add the onion and sliced asparagus and fry for 2–3 minutes until beginning to soften.

2 Add the rice and coat in the oil, then add the wine and allow it to be absorbed.

3 Bring the stock to the boil and add it to the rice mixture, ladle by ladle, allowing the liquid to be absorbed before adding any more. With the last addition of stock (which should be about 20 minutes from when you started), add the asparagus tips.

4 Once all the stock is just about absorbed, gently stir through the remaining ingredients and serve the risotto with a rocket and tomato salad.

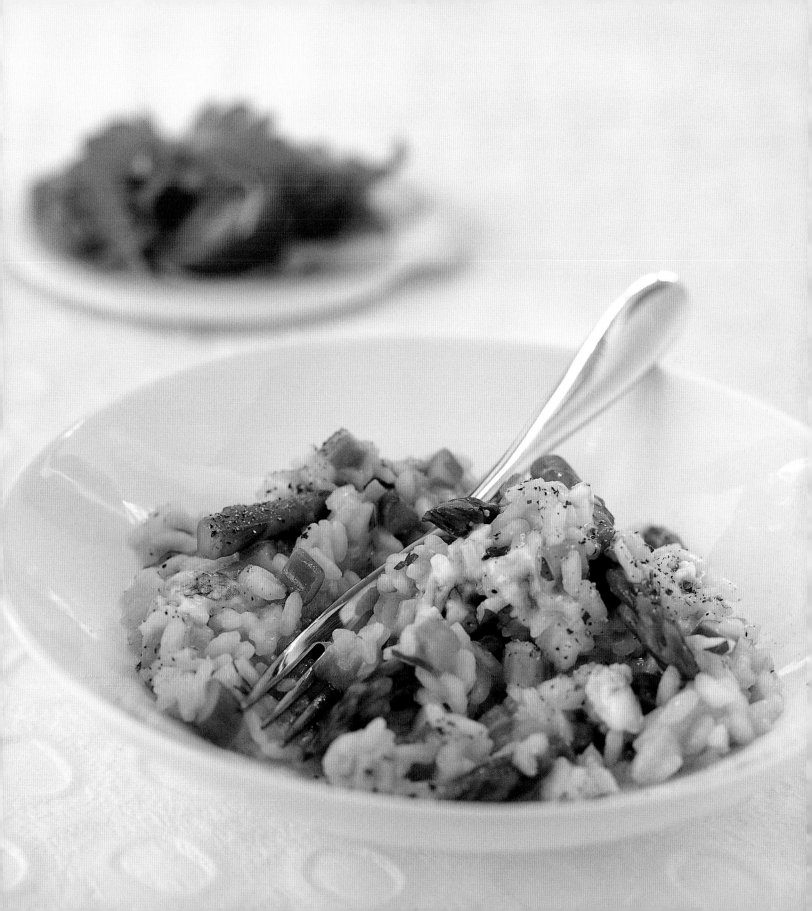

BEEF FILLET IN RED WINE
WITH PARMESAN MASH

serves 4
preparation time 10 minutes
cooking time 20 minutes

nutritional values per serving
Kcals 437 (1805 kj) Protein 30 g Carb 33 g Fat 15 g
Saturated fat 8 g Fibre 2 g

---

1 teaspoon olive oil

500 g (1 lb) beef fillet

1 onion, chopped

2 garlic cloves, crushed

1 tablespoon tomato purée

300 ml (½ pint) red wine

150 ml (¼ pint) beef stock (made with concentrated liquid stock)

3 thyme sprigs

25 g (1 oz) unsalted butter, softened

1 tablespoon plain flour

pepper

green or purple-sprouting broccoli, to serve

for the Parmesan mash

625 g (1¼ lb) potatoes

4 tablespoons light crème fraîche

4 tablespoons semi-skimmed milk

3 tablespoons freshly grated Parmesan cheese

2 tablespoons chopped chives

1 Heat the oil in a large saucepan, add the beef and fry until browned all over. Add the onion and garlic and continue to fry for 1 minute.

2 Add the tomato purée, wine, stock and thyme, then season well with pepper. Bring to the boil, then cover and simmer for 15 minutes, turning the beef occasionally.

3 Meanwhile, place the potatoes in a saucepan of boiling water and cook for 12–15 minutes until tender, then mash together with the crème fraîche, milk, Parmesan and chives.

4 Remove the beef from the pan and set aside. Mix together the butter and flour and whisk quickly into the red wine sauce, then simmer until slightly thickened.

5 Slice the beef fillet and serve with the mash and red wine sauce and some green or purple-sprouting broccoli.

SEARED TOFU

WITH STEAMED PAK CHOI

serves 4

preparation time 5 minutes, plus marinating

cooking time 5 minutes

nutritional values per serving

Kcals 115 (475 kj) Protein 10 g Carb 4 g Fat 6 g

Saturated fat 1 g Fibre 2 g

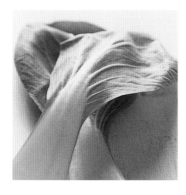

2 x 200 g (7 oz) pack tofu, cubed

2 garlic cloves, crushed

2.5-cm (1-inch) piece of fresh root
ginger, grated

2 teaspoons olive oil

1 green chilli, finely chopped (optional)

4 tablespoons oyster sauce or black bean sauce

4 pak choi, halved

basmati rice, to serve

1 Place the tofu in a non-metallic bowl with the garlic, ginger, oil and chilli, if using. Cover and leave to marinate in a cool place for 10 minutes.

2 Heat a frying pan until very hot, then add the tofu and any marinating liquid and fry quickly for 3–4 minutes until seared on all sides. Stir through the oyster or black bean sauce.

3 Meanwhile, place the pak choi in a steamer and cook for 3 minutes until just tender. Serve the tofu over the pak choi with basmati rice.

BAKED AUBERGINES
WITH FLAT BREAD AND TZATZIKI

serves 4

preparation time 10 minutes

cooking time 50 minutes

nutritional values per serving

Kcals 325 (1342 kj) Protein 11 g Carb 54 g Fat 8 g

Saturated fat 3 g Fibre 5 g

2 large aubergines, halved lengthways

1 tablespoon olive oil

100 g (3½ oz) couscous

175 ml (6 fl oz) boiling water

1 onion, finely chopped

1 garlic clove, crushed

100 g (3½ oz) ready-to-eat dried apricots, chopped

50 g (2 oz) raisins

grated rind and juice of 1 lemon

2 tablespoons chopped mint

2 tablespoons chopped coriander

2 tablespoons freshly grated Parmesan cheese

4 flat breads, to serve

for the tzatziki

½ cucumber, finely chopped

2 spring onions, sliced

200 ml (7 fl oz) light Greek yogurt

1 Place the aubergines cut-side up on a baking sheet and brush each with a little of the oil. Cook in a preheated oven, 200°C (400°F), Gas Mark 6, for 30–35 minutes until the flesh is tender, then remove (leaving the oven on) and leave to cool. When the aubergines are cool enough to touch, scoop out the flesh and roughly chop. Reserve the skins.

2 Meanwhile, place the couscous in a heatproof container, pour on the measurement water and cover with clingfilm. Set aside for 5 minutes, then remove the clingfilm and fork through.

3 Heat the remaining oil in a nonstick frying pan, add the onion and garlic and fry for 3 minutes, then stir through the apricots, raisins, lemon rind and juice, couscous, herbs, Parmesan and aubergine flesh.

4 Spoon this mixture into the aubergine skins and return them to the oven for 10 minutes.

5 Mix together the tzatziki ingredients in a serving bowl and serve with the aubergines and flat breads.

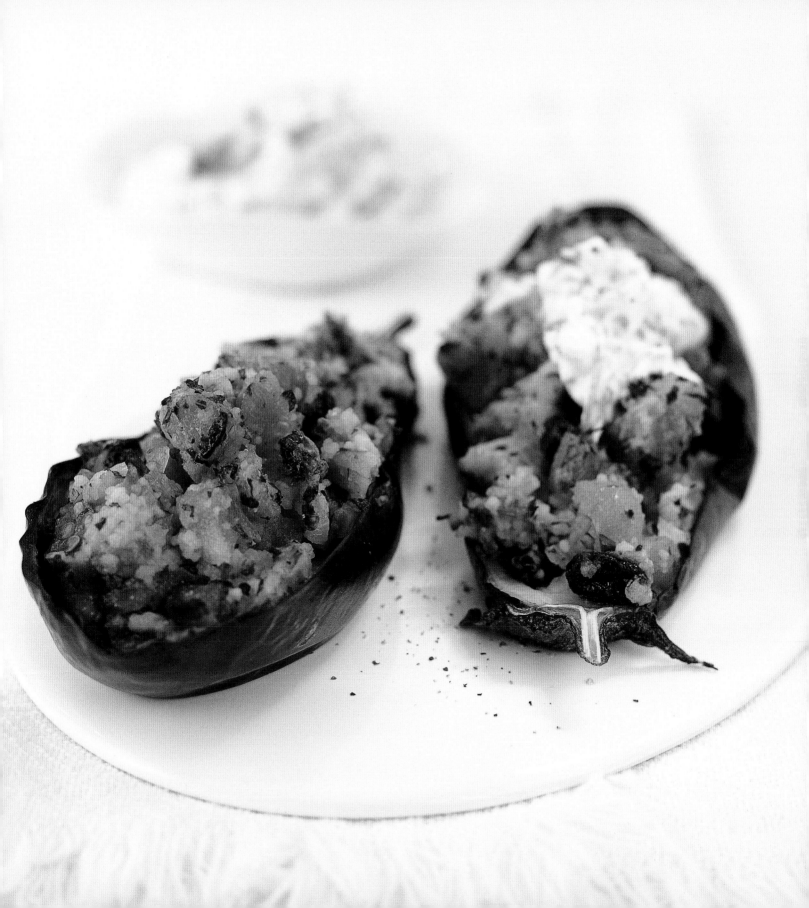

DESSERTS

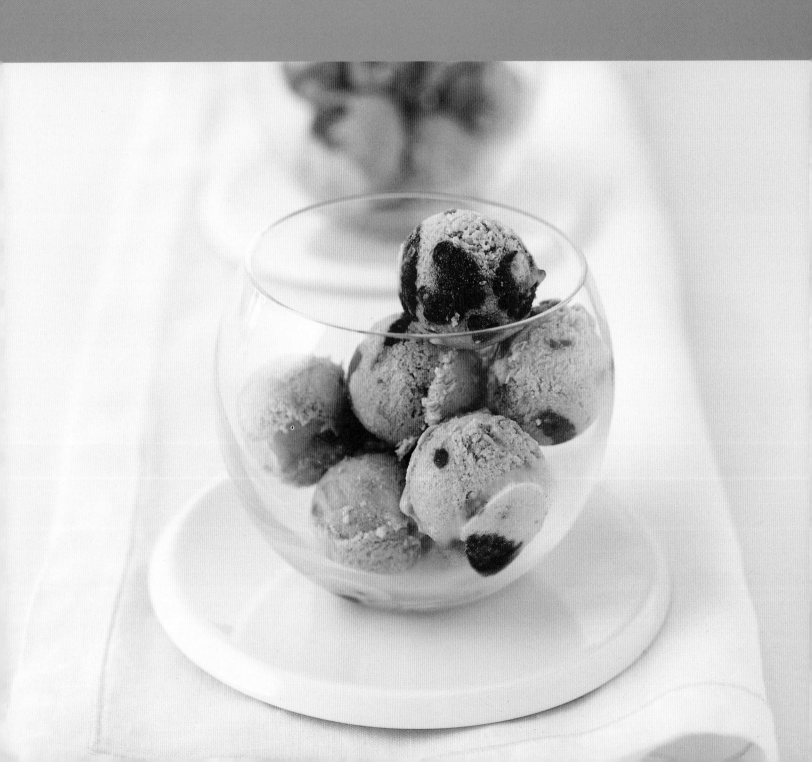

RASPBERRY AND NECTARINE
FROZEN YOGURT

serves 4
preparation time 5 minutes, plus freezing
cooking time no cooking

nutritional values per serving
Kcals 212 (869 kj) Protein 7 g Carb 28 g Fat 9 g
Saturated fat 5 g Fibre 3 g

---

300 g (10 oz) fresh or frozen raspberries

3 nectarines, peeled, stoned and cut into small pieces

2 tablespoons icing sugar

400 ml (14 fl oz) Greek yogurt

200 ml (7 fl oz) light Greek yogurt

1 Place half the raspberries and nectarines in a liquidizer or food processor and blend until smooth.

2 Stir together with the remaining ingredients, then transfer to a freezerproof container and freeze for 1 hour. Stir well, then return to the freezer and freeze until solid.

3 Serve in scoops, as you would ice cream. This will keep for up to 1 month in the freezer.

BAKED PLUMS

WITH A CRUNCHY GINGER TOPPING

serves 4

preparation time 5 minutes

cooking time 20 minutes

nutritional values per serving

Kcals 159 (657 kj) Protein 1 g Carb 23 g Fat 7 g

Saturated fat 4 g Fibre 2 g

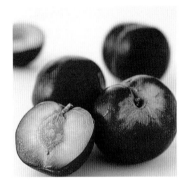

12 ripe plums, halved and stoned

6 gingernut biscuits, crumbled

25 g (1 oz) unsalted butter, melted

1 tablespoon clear honey

grated rind and juice of 1 lemon

ice cream or low-fat custard, to serve

1 Place the plums cut-sides up in a large ovenproof dish and sprinkle the biscuits over the top.

2 Mix together the remaining ingredients and drizzle over the plums. Bake in a preheated oven, 200°C (400°F), Gas Mark 6, for 15–20 minutes until the plums are tender and beginning to turn golden.

3 Serve warm with ice cream or low-fat custard.

UPSIDE-DOWN

PINEAPPLE SPONGE

serves 6

preparation time 5 minutes

cooking time 1 hour

nutritional values per serving

Kcals 277 (937 kj) Protein 4 g Carb 30 g Fat 16 g

Saturated fat 3 g Fibre 1 g

---

100 g (3½ oz) polyunsaturated margarine

100 g (3½ oz) self-raising flour, sifted

50 g (2 oz) caster sugar

2 eggs

few drops vanilla essence

1 tablespoon golden syrup

4 canned pineapple slices in juice, drained

low-fat ready-made custard or low-fat natural yogurt, to serve

1 Beat together the margarine, flour, sugar, eggs and vanilla essence in a bowl until smooth.

2 Lightly grease and flour a 600-ml (1-pint) pudding basin and spoon in the syrup. Place the pineapple slices around the bottom of the basin, then pour in the sponge mixture.

3 Cover the basin with foil, then place in a saucepan, with boiling water coming halfway up the sides of the basin, and steam for 1 hour, topping up with more boiling water as necessary.

4 Carefully lift the basin from the saucepan, remove the foil, then turn the pudding out on to a serving plate. Serve with low-fat custard or yogurt for a wonderful wintry treat.

CARAMEL PEAR

AND MARZIPAN TART

serves 8

preparation time 10 minutes

cooking time 40 minutes

nutritional values per serving

Kcals 268 (1107 kJ) Protein 2 g Carb 34 g Fat 14 g

Saturated fat 7 g Fibre 3 g

---

50 g (2 oz) unsalted butter

50 g (2 oz) soft light brown sugar

6 ripe pears, peeled, halved and cored

25 g (1 oz) marzipan

250 g (8 oz) ready-made shortcrust pastry

ice cream, to serve

1 Place the butter and sugar in a 22-cm (9-inch) fixed-bottomed cake tin. Place over a moderate heat and cook, stirring continuously, for about 5 minutes until golden.

2 Stuff a little marzipan into the cavity of each pear half, then carefully arrange them cut-side up in the tin.

3 Roll out the pastry on a lightly floured surface to the size of the tin, then place over the top of the pears and press down all around them. Bake in a preheated oven, 190°C (375°F), Gas Mark 5, for about 40 minutes until the pastry is golden and the juices are bubbling.

4 Cool in the tin for 10 minutes, then invert on to a large plate and serve with a little ice cream.

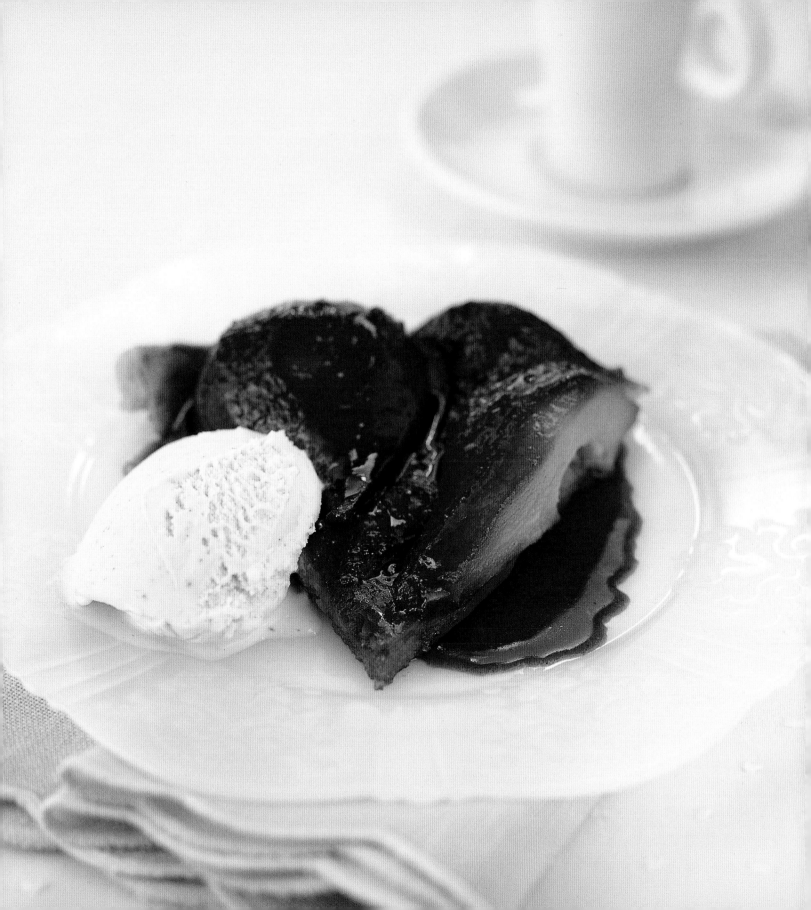

SPICED ORANGE

RICE PUDDING

serves 4

preparation time 5 minutes

cooking time 20 minutes

nutritional values per serving

Kcals 295 (1218 kj) Protein 10 g Carb 44 g Fat 10 g

Saturated fat 2 g Fibre 1 g

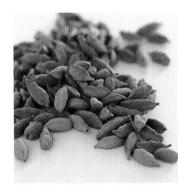

1 Place all the ingredients, except the orange segments, in a medium saucepan, bring to the boil and simmer gently for 20 minutes until the rice is tender and the milk absorbed.

2 Stir through the orange segments and serve.

900 ml (1½ pints) semi-skimmed milk

125 g (4 oz) short-grain pudding rice

2 tablespoons caster sugar

pinch of grated nutmeg

4 cardamom pods, split

grated rind and segments of 2 oranges

10-MINUTE

BLACK FOREST TRIFLES

serves 4

preparation time 10 minutes, plus chilling

cooking time no cooking

nutritional values per serving

Kcals 214 (883 kj) Protein 4 g Carb 39 g Fat 5 g

Saturated fat 4 g Fibre 1 g

---

400 g (13 oz) can black cherries in juice, drained and juice reserved

1 tablespoon kirsch

100 g (3½ oz) amaretti biscuits, halved

½ x 400 g (13 oz) carton low-fat ready-made custard

4 tablespoons light crème fraîche

25 g (1 oz) plain dark chocolate, grated

1 Divide the cherries between 4 tall glasses. Stir together 3 tablespoons of the reserved cherry juice with the kirsch.

2 Place the amaretti biscuits on top of the cherries, then pour over the juice mixture.

3 Spoon over the custard, then top with crème fraîche. Finally, sprinkle over the grated chocolate. Chill for 30 minutes, then serve.

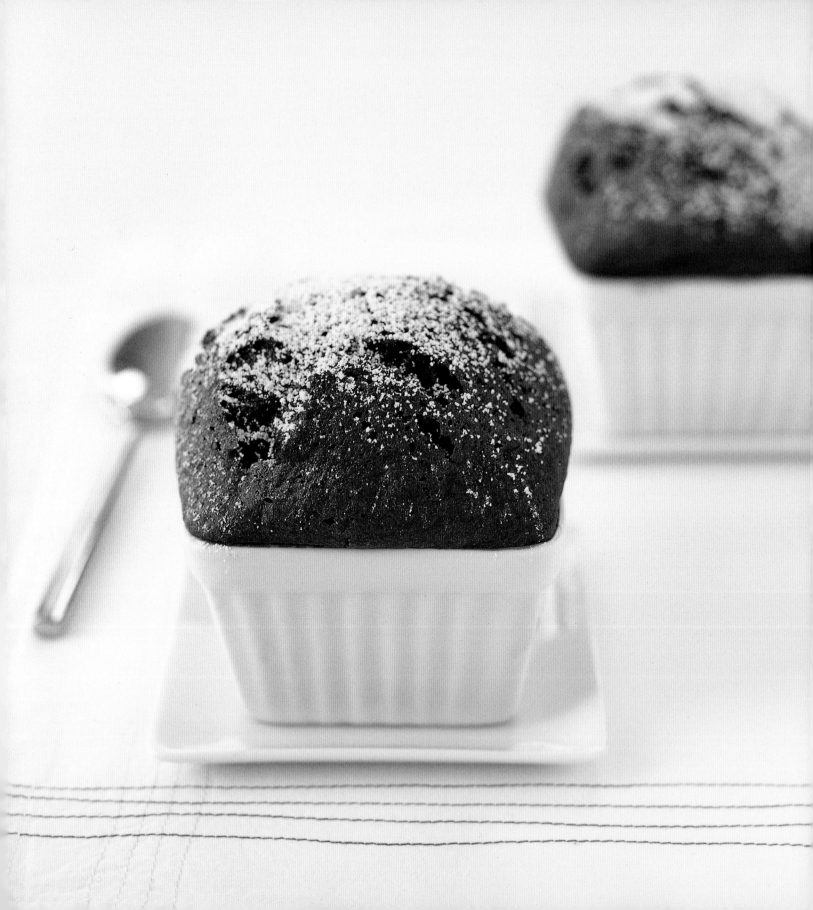

CHOCOLATE AND RASPBERRY
SOUFFLÉS

serves 4

preparation time 10 minutes

cooking time 15 minutes

nutritional values per serving

Kcals 287 (1185 kj) Protein 8 g Carb 38 g Fat 12 g

Saturated fat 6 g Fibre 1 g

---

100 g (3½ oz) plain dark chocolate

3 eggs, separated

50 g (2 oz) self-raising flour, sifted

40 g (1½ oz) caster sugar

150 g (5 oz) raspberries

to serve

icing sugar

raspberries (optional)

1 Break the chocolate into squares and place in a heatproof bowl over a saucepan of simmering water, then leave until melted.

2 Place the melted chocolate in a large bowl and whisk in the egg yolks. Fold in the flour.

3 Whisk the egg whites and caster sugar in a medium bowl until they form soft peaks. Beat a spoonful of the egg whites into the chocolate mixture to loosen it up before gently folding in the rest.

4 Divide the raspberries between 4 lightly greased ramekins, pour over the chocolate mixture, then bake in a preheated oven, 190°C (375°F), Gas Mark 5, for 12–15 minutes until the soufflés have risen.

5 Sprinkle with icing sugar and serve with extra raspberries, if desired.

SPICED FRUIT
AND NUT SALAD

serves 4

preparation time 5 minutes, plus cooling

cooking time 5 minutes

nutritional values per serving

Kcals 311 (1284 kj) Protein 8 g Carb 48 g Fat 11 g

Saturated fat 1 g Fibre 11 g

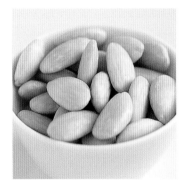

1 Place all the ingredients in a medium saucepan, bring to the boil, then remove from the heat and set aside to cool for at least 30 minutes.

2 Serve with light Greek yogurt or crème fraîche.

500 g (1 lb) mixed dried fruit, e.g., figs, apricots, prunes and papayas

75 g (3 oz) blanched almonds

300 ml (½ pint) strong black Earl Grey tea

150 ml (¼ pint) apple juice

2 star anise

6 cardamom pods

1 cinnamon stick

4 cloves

light Greek yogurt or crème fraîche, to serve

CHERRY CLAFOUTIS
WITH FLAKED ALMONDS

serves 6

preparation time 10 minutes

cooking time 50 minutes

nutritional values per serving

Kcals 252 (1040 kj) Protein 9 g Carb 41 g Fat 7 g

Saturated fat 2 g Fibre 2 g

---

500 g (1 lb) cherries, stoned

125 g (4 oz) plain flour, sifted

75 g (3 oz) caster sugar

3 eggs, beaten

400 ml (14 fl oz) semi-skimmed milk

25 g (1 oz) flaked almonds

whipping cream or low-fat ready-made
custard, to serve

1 Place the cherries in a lightly greased 1-litre (1¾-pint) baking dish.

2 Place the flour in a bowl and stir in the sugar. Make a well in the centre and pour in the eggs and milk. Gradually beat the flour mixture into the liquid, drawing it in from the side, to make a smooth batter, then pour this over the cherries.

3 Sprinkle over the flaked almonds, then bake in a preheated oven, 180°C (350°F), Gas Mark 4, for 45–50 minutes until just firm and golden. Serve with a little whipping cream or low-fat custard.

ST CLEMENTS

CHEESECAKE

serves 10

preparation time 10 minutes, plus cooling and chilling

cooking time 50 minutes

nutritional values per serving

Kcals 194 (801 kj) Protein 10 g Carb 19 g Fat 9 g

Saturated fat 4 g Fibre 1 g

---

50 g (2 oz) unsalted butter

175 g (6 oz) low-fat oat biscuits, crushed

2 x 250 g (8 oz) tubs Quark

125 g (4 oz) caster sugar

2 eggs

grated rind and juice of 2 oranges

grated rind and juice of 1 lemon

75 g (3 oz) sultanas

juliennes of orange and lemon rind,
to decorate

1 Lightly grease a 20-cm (8-inch) nonstick loose-bottomed round cake tin.

2 Melt the butter in a saucepan, stir in the biscuit crumbs, then press them over the base and side of the cake tin. Bake in a preheated oven, 150°C (300°F), Gas Mark 2, for 10 minutes.

3 Beat together the remaining ingredients in a bowl, spoon them into the cake tin and bake for 40 minutes until just firm. Turn off the oven and leave the cheesecake to cool for an hour in the oven.

4 Chill for 2 hours, then serve decorated with juliennes of orange and lemon rind.

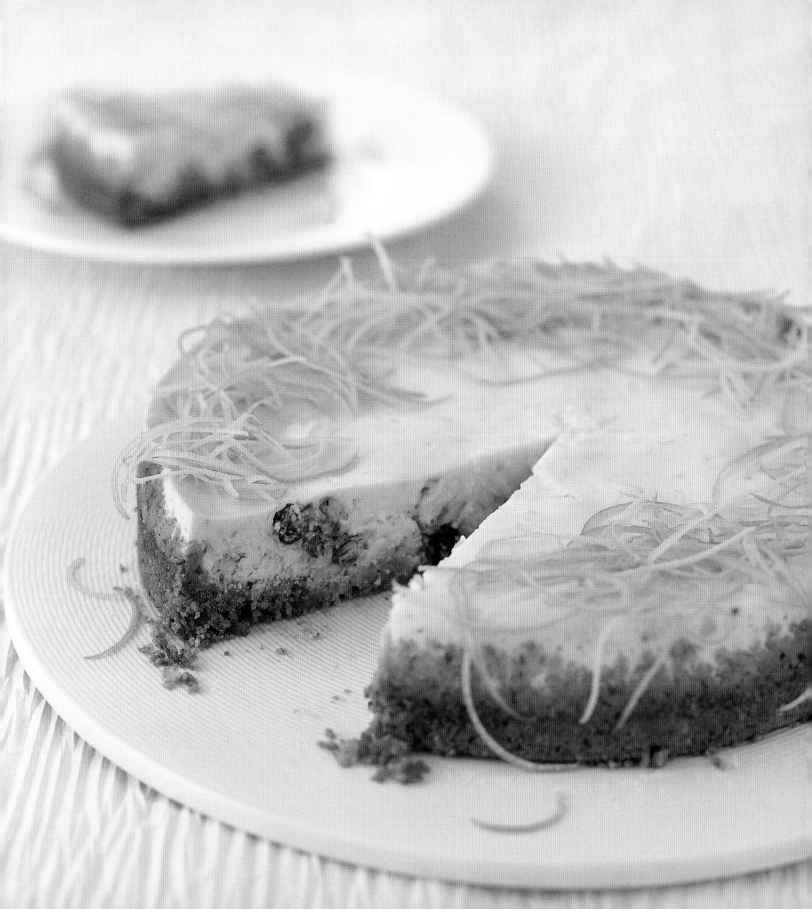

BANANA AND PECAN PANCAKES
WITH MAPLE SYRUP

serves 4 (makes 8 pancakes)
preparation time 5 minutes
cooking time 5 minutes

nutritional values per serving
Kcals 292 (1206 kj) Protein 8 g Carb 51 g Fat 7 g
Saturated fat 1 g Fibre 2 g

---

150 g (5 oz) self-raising flour

1 tablespoon baking powder

1 tablespoon caster sugar

½ teaspoon ground cinnamon

1 large egg, beaten

200 ml (7 fl oz) semi-skimmed milk

olive oil, for frying

2 bananas, sliced

25 g (1 oz) pecan nuts, toasted and chopped

2 tablespoons maple syrup

1 Sift together the flour and baking powder in a bowl, then stir in the sugar and cinnamon. Make a well in the centre.

2 Mix together the egg and milk, then pour into the well. Gradually beat the flour mixture into the liquid, drawing it in from the side, to make a thick smooth batter.

3 Brush a large nonstick frying pan with a little oil. Place a tablespoonful of the mixture in the pan, tilting the pan to coat the base, and cook for 1 minute on each side until golden, then remove the pancake and keep warm. Repeat with the remaining batter.

4 Top the pancakes with banana slices and chopped pecans, and drizzle over the maple syrup.

BAKED PEARS
WITH ALMOND MERINGUE

serves 4

preparation time 5 minutes

cooking time 20 minutes

nutritional values per serving

Kcals 260 (1074 kj) Protein 6 g Carb 61 g Fat 11 g

Saturated fat 1 g Fibre 5 g

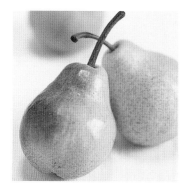

4 ripe pears, peeled, halved and cored

2 egg whites

75 g (3 oz) caster sugar

75 g (3 oz) ground almonds

light crème fraîche or ice cream, to serve

1 Place the pears in an ovenproof dish.

2 Whisk the egg whites in a medium bowl until they form stiff peaks. Whisk in the sugar and ground almonds, then spoon this over the pear halves.

3 Bake in a preheated oven, 180°C (350°F), Gas Mark 4, for 15–20 minutes until golden. Serve with light crème fraîche or ice cream.

CHOCOLATE BRIOCHE
PUDDING

serves 4

preparation time 10 minutes

cooking time 30 minutes

nutritional values per serving

Kcals 287 (1185 kj) Protein 4 g Carb 61 g Fat 10 g

Saturated fat 3 g Fibre 0 g

---

15 g (½ oz) unsalted butter

75 g (3 oz) plain dark chocolate

1 tablespoon caster sugar

300 ml (½ pint) semi-skimmed milk

2 large eggs

3 brioche rolls, each cut into 4 slices

light crème fraîche, to serve

1 Lightly grease a shallow ovenproof dish measuring 18 x 23 cm (7 x 9 inches).

2 Place the butter, chocolate, sugar and milk in a small saucepan and heat gently until the sugar has dissolved and the chocolate has melted. Set aside to cool a little.

3 Whisk the eggs in a medium bowl, then gradually add the chocolate mixture, whisking continuously. Soak each slice of brioche in the chocolate mixture, then layer them into the dish.

4 Pour over any excess liquid, then cook in a preheated oven, 200°C (400°F), Gas Mark 6, for 25–30 minutes until risen and just set. Serve with light crème fraîche.

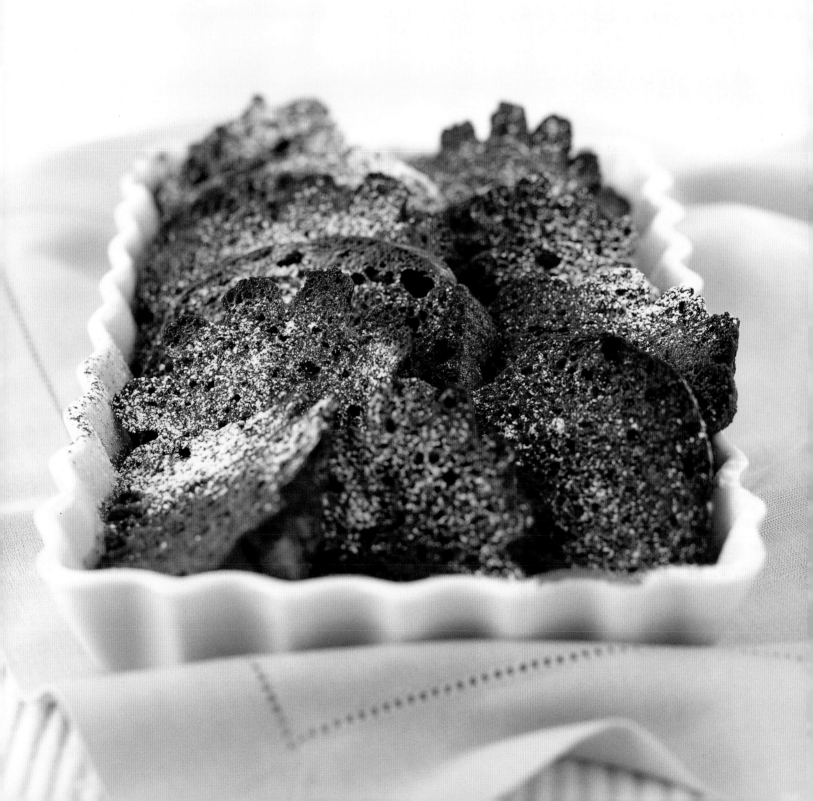

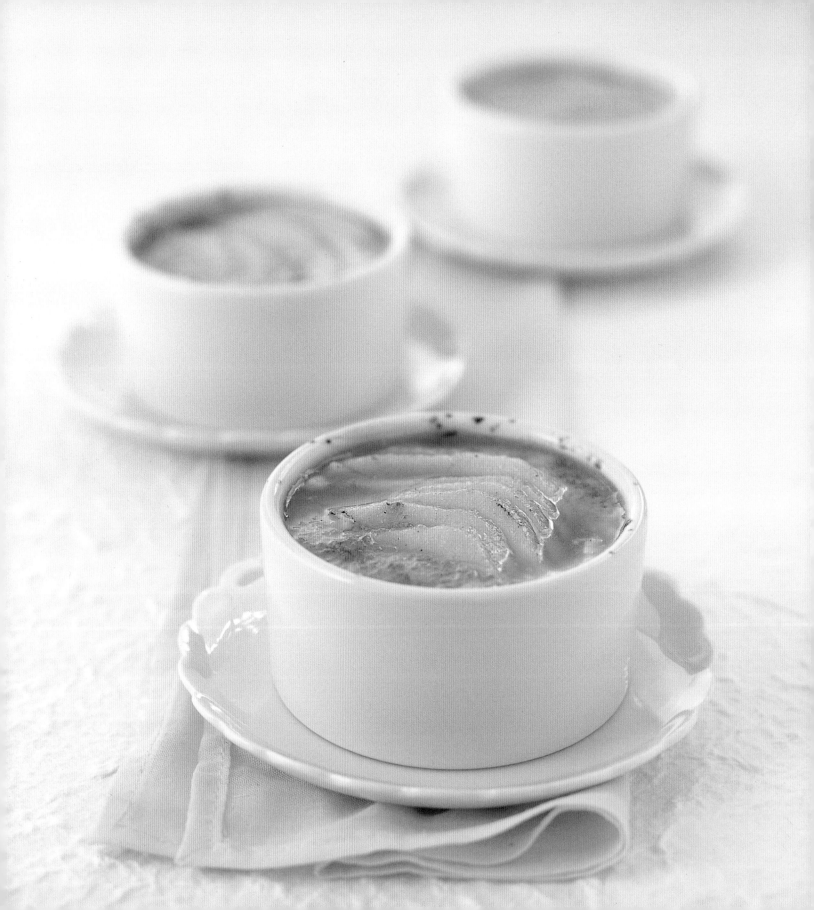

CHEAT'S MANGO
AND PASSION FRUIT BRÛLÉE

serves 4

preparation time 10 minutes, plus chilling

cooking time 2 minutes

nutritional values per serving

Kcals 131 (541 kj) Protein 5 g Carb 19 g Fat 5 g

Saturated fat 4 g Fibre 1 g

---

1 small mango, peeled, stoned and thinly sliced

2 passion fruit, flesh scooped out

300 g (10 oz) low-fat natural yogurt

200 g (7 oz) light crème fraîche

1 tablespoon icing sugar

few drops vanilla essence

2 tablespoons demerara sugar

1 Divide the mango slices between 4 ramekins.

2 Stir together the passion fruit flesh, yogurt, crème fraîche, icing sugar and vanilla essence in a bowl, then spoon over the mango. Tap each ramekin to level the surface.

3 Sprinkle over the demerara sugar and cook under a high grill for 1–2 minutes until the sugar has melted. Chill for about 30 minutes, then serve.

ORANGE, RHUBARB
AND GINGER SLUMP

serves 6

preparation time 10 minutes

cooking time 15 minutes

nutritional values per serving

Kcals 278 (1148 kj) Protein 4 g Carb 32 g Fat 15 g

Saturated fat 10 g Fibre 3 g

---

750 g (1½ lb) rhubarb, chopped into 1.5-cm (¾-inch) pieces

½ teaspoon ground ginger

50 g (2 oz) golden caster sugar

grated rind and juice of 1 orange

4 tablespoons mascarpone cheese

175 g (6 oz) self-raising flour, sifted

50 g (2 oz) unsalted butter, cut into small pieces

grated rind of ½ lemon

6 tablespoons semi-skimmed milk

low-fat ready-made custard, to serve

1 Place the rhubarb, ginger, half the sugar and orange rind and juice in a medium saucepan. Bring to the boil and simmer gently for 5–6 minutes until the rhubarb is just tender.

2 Transfer the rhubarb to an ovenproof dish and spoon over dollops of mascarpone.

3 Place the flour in a bowl. Add the butter and rub in with the fingertips until the mixture resembles fine breadcrumbs. Quickly stir through the remaining sugar, the lemon rind and milk until combined. Place spoonfuls of the mixture over the rhubarb and mascarpone.

4 Cook in a preheated oven, 200°C (400°F), Gas Mark 6, for 12–15 minutes until golden and bubbling. Serve with low-fat custard.

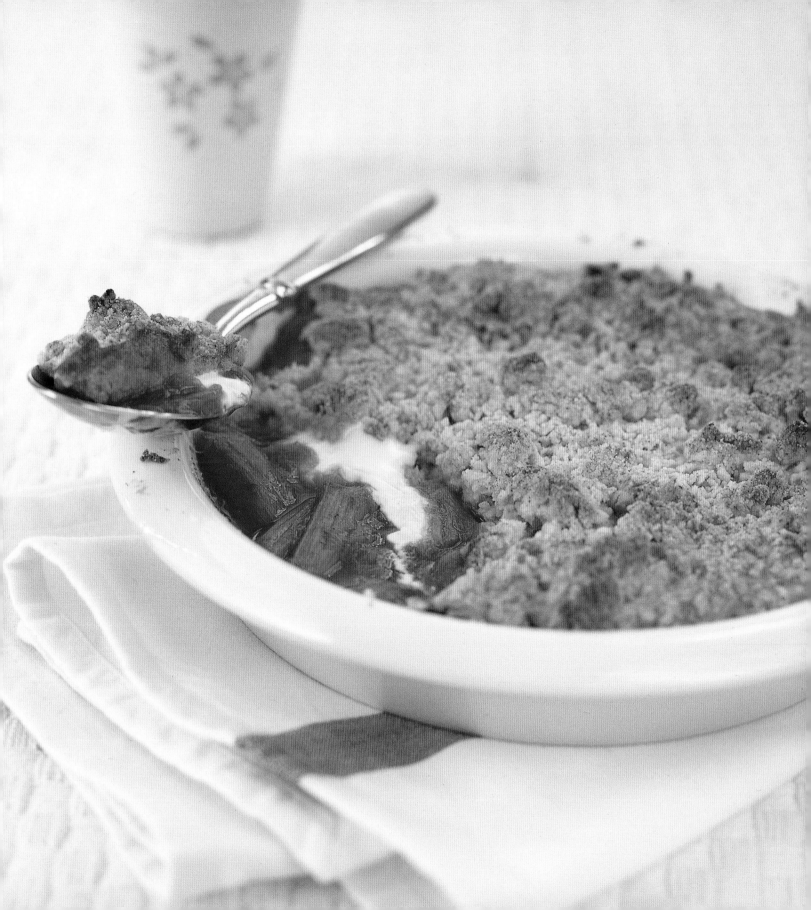

RASPBERRY

SHORTCAKE MESS

serves 4

preparation time 5 minutes

cooking time no cooking

nutritional values per serving

Kcals 260 (1073 kj) Protein 9 g Carb 30 g Fat 12 g

Saturated fat 8 g Fibre 2 g

300 g (10 oz) raspberries, roughly crushed

4 shortbread fingers, roughly crushed

400 g (13 oz) 8 per cent fat fromage frais

2 tablespoons icing sugar or artificial sweetener

1 Gently combine all the ingredients, reserving a few of the raspberries for decoration, in a bowl. Divide between 4 serving dishes.

2 Serve immediately, decorated with the reserved raspberries.

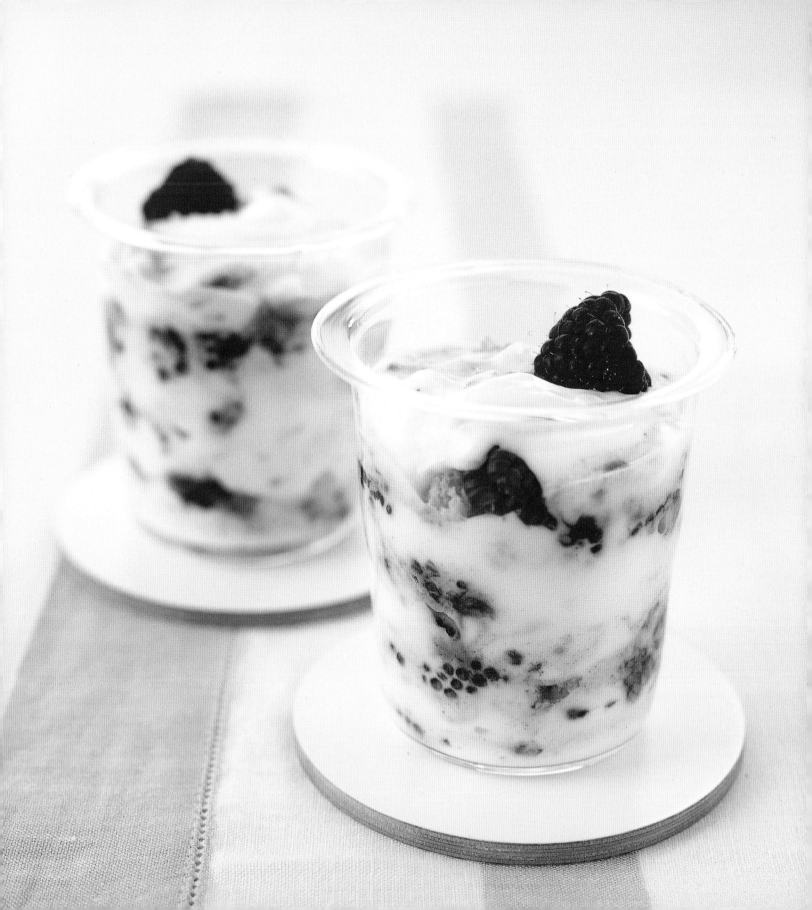

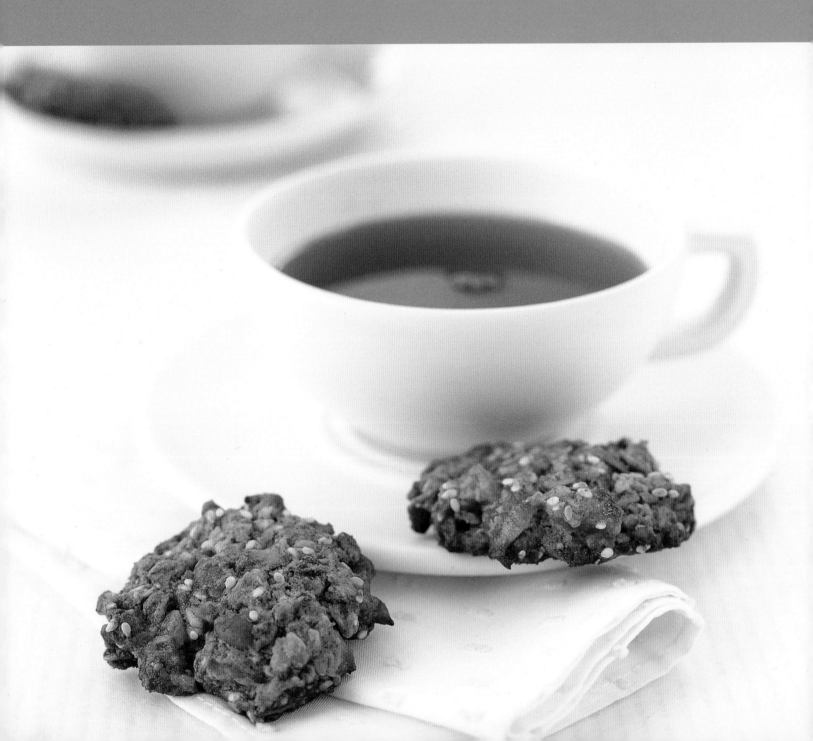

BAKING

APRICOT, FIG
AND MIXED-SEED BITES

makes 24
preparation time 10 minutes
cooking time 15 minutes

nutritional values per bite
Kcals 107 (449 kj) Protein 2 g Carb 10 g Fat 7 g
Saturated fat 1 g Fibre 1 g

---

150 g (5 oz) polyunsaturated margarine

75 g (3 oz) soft light brown sugar

1 egg, beaten

2 tablespoons water

75 g (3 oz) plain wholemeal flour

½ teaspoon bicarbonate of soda

100 g (3½ oz) rolled oats

50 g (2 oz) ready-to-eat dried apricots, chopped

50 g (2 oz) dried figs, chopped

50 g (2 oz) mixed seeds, e.g., pumpkin, sunflower and sesame

1 Beat together the margarine and sugar in a bowl until light and fluffy, then beat in the egg and measurement water.

2 Sift together the flour and bicarbonate of soda into the bowl, adding any bran in the sieve. Add the oats, apricots, figs and seeds, then fold all the ingredients into the margarine and sugar mixture.

3 Place walnut-sized pieces of the mixture on baking sheets lined with greaseproof paper or baking parchment and flatten them slightly with the back of a fork.

4 Bake in a preheated oven, 180°C (350°F), Gas Mark 4, for 10–15 minutes until golden. Transfer to a wire rack to cool. These bites may be stored for up to 2 days in an airtight container.

COOKIES

WITH THREE FLAVOURS

makes 30

preparation time 10 minutes

cooking time 6 minutes

nutritional values per serving

Kcals 60/61/60 (251/255/251 kj) Protein 1/1/1 g Carb 9/9/9 g

Fat 4/4/4 g Saturated fat 1/1/1 g Fibre 0/0/0 g

---

50 g (2 oz) unsalted butter, softened, or
polyunsaturated margarine

40 g (1½ oz) granulated sugar

25 g (1 oz) soft light brown sugar

1 egg, beaten

few drops of vanilla essence

150 g (5 oz) self-raising flour, sifted

50 g (2 oz) rolled oats

Flavours

50 g (2 oz) dried cranberries
40 g (1½ oz) hazelnuts, toasted and chopped

40 g (1½ oz) pistachios nuts, chopped
40 g (1½ oz) dried banana chips, chopped

2 pieces of stem ginger, chopped
½ teaspoon grated fresh root ginger
40 g (1½ oz) plain dark chocolate drops

1 Beat together the butter, sugars, egg and vanilla essence in a large bowl until smooth.

2 Stir in the flour and oats, then add the flavours of your choice (see below).

3 Place teaspoonfuls of the mixture on to baking sheets lined with greaseproof paper or baking parchment and flatten them slightly with the back of a fork.

4 Bake in a preheated oven, 180°C (350°F), Gas Mark 4, for about 5–6 minutes until browned. Transfer to a wire rack to cool. These cookies may be stored for up to 2 days in an airtight container.

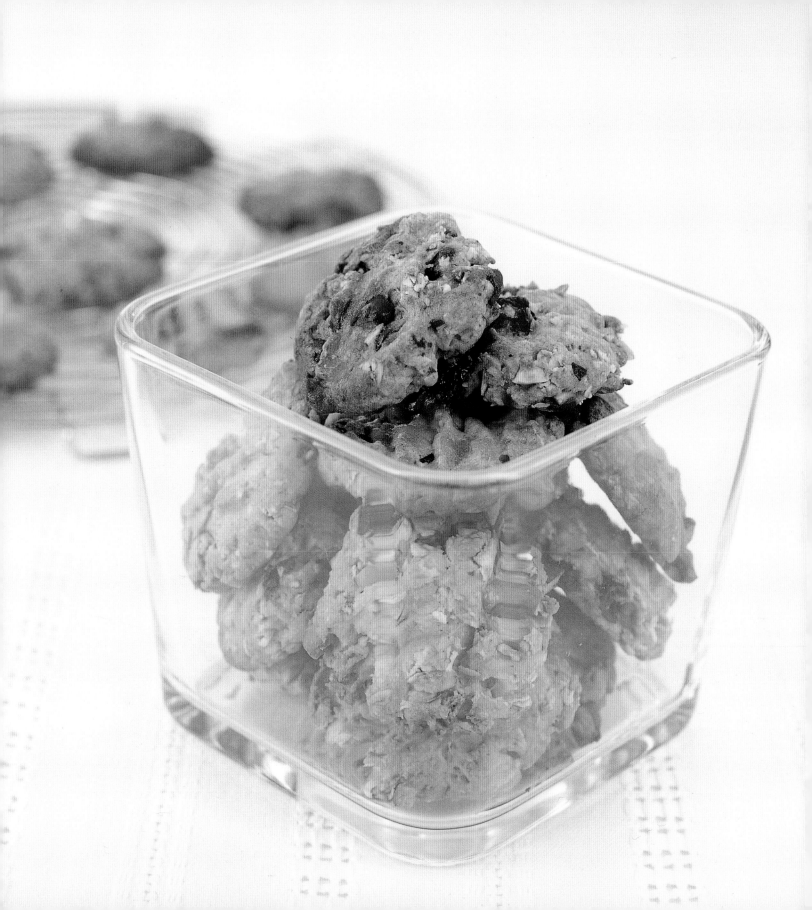

MINIATURE ORANGE
SHORTBREADS

makes 80
preparation time 10 minutes
cooking time 12 minutes

nutritional values per shortbread

Kcals 30 (123 kj) Protein 00 g Carb 3 g Fat 2 g
Saturated fat 1 g Fibre 0 g

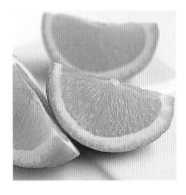

250 g (8 oz) plain flour, sifted

**175 g (6 oz) unsalted butter, cut into
small pieces**

grated rind of 1 orange

½ teaspoon mixed spice

75 g (3 oz) caster sugar

2 teaspoons cold water

to serve

2 teaspoons icing sugar

1 teaspoon cocoa powder

1 Place the flour in a bowl, add the butter and rub in with the fingertips until the mixture resembles fine breadcrumbs. Stir in the remaining ingredients with the measurement water and mix to form a dough.

2 Roll out on a lightly floured surface to a thickness of 2.5 mm (⅛ inch). Using a 1.5-cm (¾-inch) plain cutter, cut out approximately 80 rounds.

3 Place the rounds on nonstick baking sheets and bake in a preheated oven, 200°C (400°F), Gas Mark 6, for 10–12 minutes until golden. Carefully transfer to a wire rack to cool.

4 Mix together the icing sugar and cocoa powder and dust a little over the biscuits before serving. These shortbreads are best eaten on the same day.

BAKED FRUIT, NUT
AND SEED BARS

makes 16
preparation time 10 minutes
cooking time 50 minutes

nutritional values per bar
Kcals 116 (479 kj) Protein 2 g Carb 16 g Fat 5 g
Saturated fat 1 g Fibre 2 g

---

500 g (1 lb) pears, peeled, cored and chopped

½ teaspoon ground cinnamon

5 tablespoons apple juice

250 g (8 oz) dates, chopped

50 g (2 oz) walnuts, chopped

75 g (3 oz) self-raising flour, sifted

25 g (1 oz) ground almonds

40 g (1½ oz) mixed seeds, e.g., sunflower and pumpkin

1 tablespoon unsalted butter, softened, or polyunsaturated margarine

1 Place the pears, cinnamon and apple juice in a saucepan and bring to the boil. Cover and simmer for 8–10 minutes until really soft, then mash the pears and liquid until smooth.

2 Stir all the remaining ingredients into the mashed pears, then spoon the mixture into a greased and lined 20-cm (8-inch) square baking tin.

3 Bake in a preheated oven, 200°C (400°F), Gas Mark 6, for 30–40 minutes until golden and firm to touch. Mark into 16 squares, then cool in the tin for 10 minutes before transferring to a wire rack. These bars may be stored for up to 2 days in an airtight container.

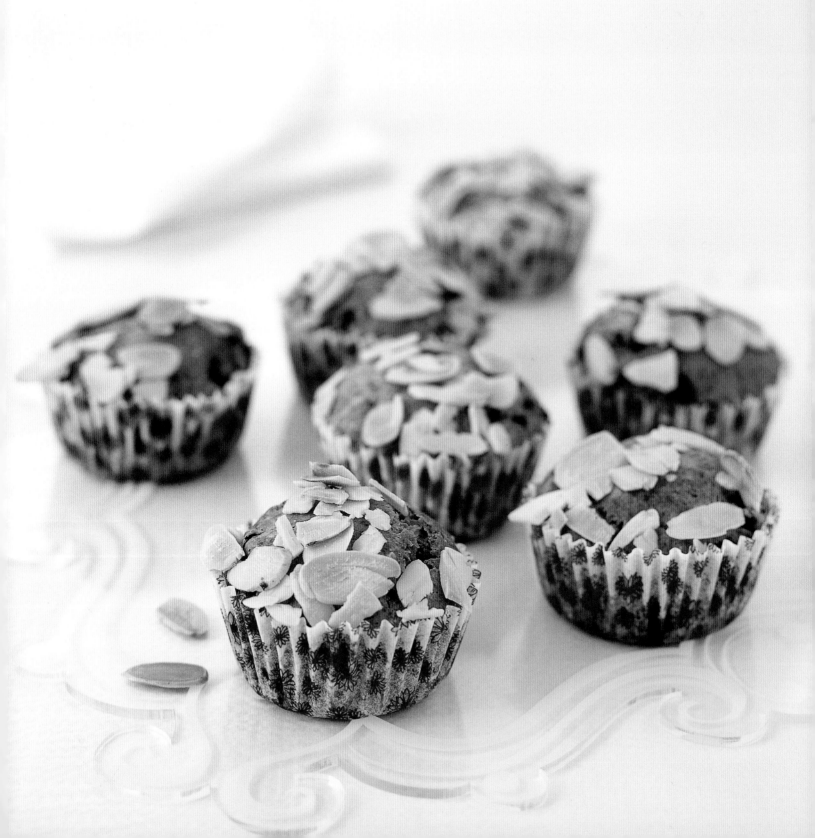

BLACKCURRANT
AND ALMOND MUFFINS

makes 12
preparation time 5 minutes
cooking time 25 minutes

nutritional values per muffin
Kcals 153 (632 kj) Protein 3 g Carb 20 g Fat 7 g
Saturated fat 4 g Fibre 1 g

200 g (7 oz) plain flour

2 teaspoons baking powder

½ teaspoon bicarbonate of soda

pinch of salt

50 g (2 oz) caster sugar

few drops of almond essence

75 g (3 oz) unsalted butter, melted

200 ml (7 fl oz) buttermilk

300 g (10 oz) can blackcurrants in natural juice, drained, or 250 g (8 oz) fresh or frozen blackcurrants

40 g (1½ oz) flaked almonds

1 Sift together the flour, baking powder, bicarbonate of soda and salt into a bowl, then stir in the sugar.

2 Mix together the almond essence, melted butter, buttermilk and blackcurrants in a separate large bowl, then very lightly stir in the dry ingredients. The mixture should still look a little lumpy.

3 Spoon the mixture into a 12-cup muffin tin lined with muffin cases, sprinkle over the flaked almonds, then bake in a preheated oven, 190°C (375°F), Gas Mark 5, for 20–25 minutes until risen and golden. Carefully lift the cases from the tin and transfer to a wire rack to cool. These muffins are best eaten on the same day.

LAYERED RHUBARB

TRAY BAKES

makes 8

preparation time 10 minutes

cooking time 15 minutes

nutritional values per bake

Kcals 157 (648 kj) Protein 3 g Carb 20 g Fat 8 g

Saturated fat 1 g Fibre 2 g

---

50 g (2 oz) polyunsaturated margarine

2 tablespoons golden syrup

1 tablespoon soft light brown sugar

75 g (3 oz) rolled oats

50 g (2 oz) self-raising wholemeal flour, sifted

pinch ground ginger

25 g (1 oz) pecan nuts, chopped

6 tablespoons rhubarb compote or stewed rhubarb

1 Place the margarine, syrup and sugar in a saucepan and heat gently until the sugar has dissolved. Stir in the oats, flour, ginger and pecans and combine well.

2 Spoon two-thirds of the mixture into a 15-cm (6-inch) nonstick square baking tin and gently press down. Spoon over the rhubarb, then sprinkle over the remaining oat mixture and press down lightly.

3 Bake in a preheated oven, 180°C (350°F), Gas Mark 4, for 15 minutes until golden. Cool in the tin, marking the mixture into 8 rectangles while still warm. These bakes are best eaten on the same day.

APPLE AND PLUM CAKE
WITH FLAKED ALMONDS

serves 12

preparation time 10 minutes

cooking time 1 hour

nutritional values per serving

Kcals 217 (896 kj) Protein 3 g Carb 35 g Fat 8 g

Saturated fat 5 g Fibre 1 g

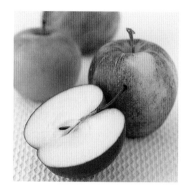

250 g (8 oz) plain flour

2 teaspoons baking powder

175 g (6 oz) caster sugar

3 eggs

grated rind of 1 orange

100 g (3½ oz) unsalted butter or polyunsaturated margarine, melted

2 tablespoons semi-skimmed milk

2 dessert apples, peeled, cored and chopped

8 plums, stoned and chopped

25 g (1 oz) flaked almonds

low-fat Greek yogurt, to serve (optional)

1 Sift together the flour and baking powder into a bowl. Whisk together the sugar and eggs in a separate bowl until pale and thick.

2 Gently fold the flour mixture, orange rind, butter or margarine and milk into the egg mixture, then pour into a lightly greased and lined 23-cm (9-inch) round cake tin. Scatter the fruit and flaked almonds over the top of the cake (much of the fruit will sink into the mixture).

3 Bake in a preheated oven, 180°C (350°F), Gas Mark 4, for 1 hour until firm to touch. Leave to cool a little in the tin, then transfer to a wire rack.

4 Serve warm or cold. If you want to turn this cake into a special dessert, serve with some low-fat Greek yogurt. This cake may be stored for up to 2 days in an airtight container.

MOIST BANANA

AND CARROT CAKE

serves 14

preparation time 10 minutes

cooking time 1 hour 40 minutes

nutritional values per serving

Kcals 183 (756 kj) Protein 4 g Carb 27 g Fat 8 g

Saturated fat 1 g Fibre 2 g

---

175 g (6 oz) ready-to-eat dried apricots,
roughly chopped

125 ml (4 fl oz) water

1 egg

2 tablespoons clear honey

100 g (3½ oz) walnuts, roughly chopped

500 g (1 lb) ripe bananas, mashed

1 large carrot, about 125 g (4 oz), grated

225 g (7½ oz) self-raising flour, sifted

for the topping

150 g (5 oz) extra-light cream cheese

2 tablespoons lemon curd

1 Place the apricots in a small saucepan with the measurement water, bring to the boil and simmer for 10 minutes, then transfer to a liquidizer or food processor and blend to give a thick purée.

2 Place all the other cake ingredients in a large bowl and add the apricot purée. Mix well, then spoon into a greased and lined 1-kg (2-lb) loaf tin.

3 Bake in a preheated oven, 180°C (350°F), Gas Mark 4, for 1½ hours or until a skewer inserted in the middle comes out clean. Turn out on to a wire rack to cool.

4 Beat together the cream cheese and lemon curd and spread over the top of the loaf. This loaf may be stored for up to 2–3 days in the fridge.

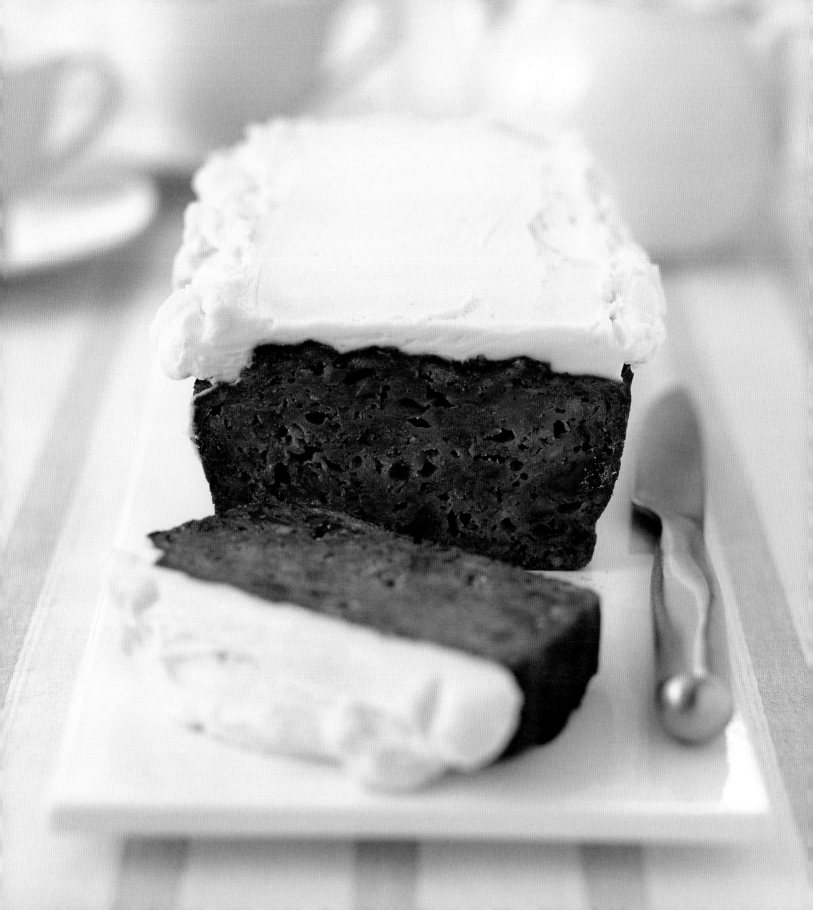

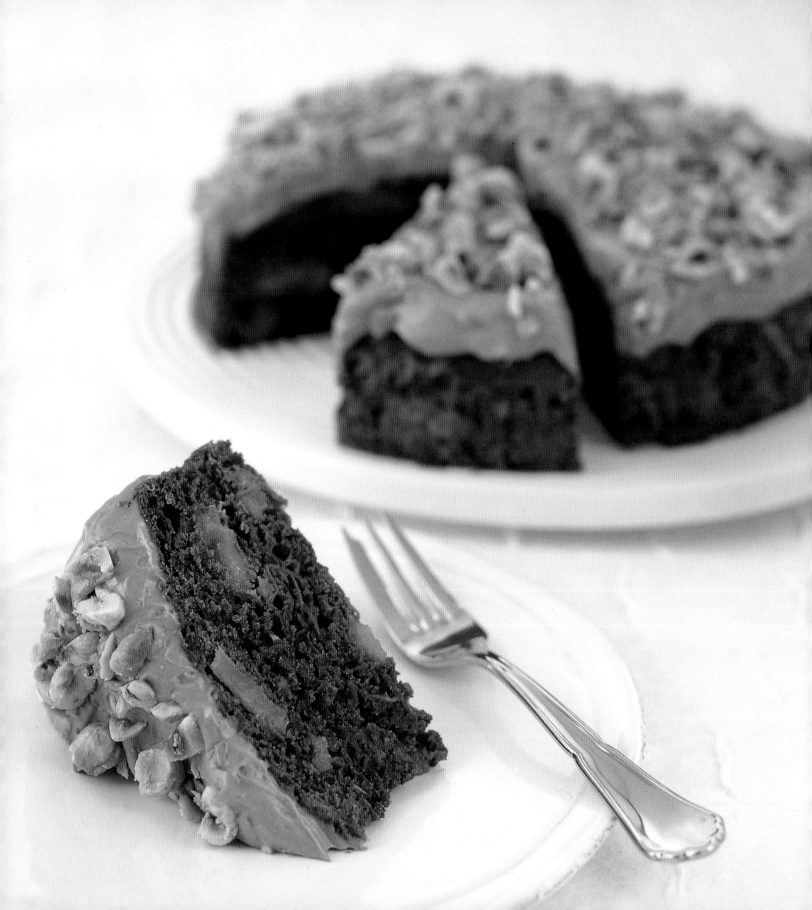

CHOCOLATE, COURGETTE
AND NUT CAKE

serves 12

preparation time 10 minutes

cooking time 40 minutes

nutritional values per serving

Kcals 266 (1099 kj) Protein 4 g Carb 30 g Fat 11 g

Saturated fat 2 g Fibre 1 g

---

250 g (8 oz) courgettes, coarsely grated

2 eggs

100 ml (3½ fl oz) vegetable oil

grated rind and juice of 1 orange

125 g (4 oz) caster sugar

225 g (7½ oz) self-raising flour

2 tablespoons cocoa powder

½ teaspoon bicarbonate of soda

½ teaspoon baking powder

50 g (2 oz) ready-to-eat dried apricots,
chopped

for the topping

200 g (7 oz) extra-light cream cheese

2 tablespoons chocolate hazelnut spread

1 tablespoon hazelnuts, toasted and chopped

1 Place the courgettes in a sieve and squeeze out any excess liquid.

2 Beat together the eggs, oil, orange rind and juice and sugar in a large bowl. Sift in the flour, cocoa powder, bicarbonate of soda and baking powder and beat to combine.

3 Fold in the courgettes and apricots, then spoon the mixture into a greased and lined 20-cm (8-in) deep loose-bottomed cake tin.

4 Bake in a preheated oven, 180°C (350°F), Gas Mark 4, for 40 minutes until risen and firm to touch. Turn out on to a wire rack to cool.

5 Beat together the cream cheese and chocolate hazelnut spread and spread over the top of the cake. Sprinkle over the hazelnuts. This cake may be stored for up to 2–3 days in an airtight container.

PARMESAN

AND HERB SCONES

makes 12

preparation time 10 minutes

cooking time 12 minutes

nutritional values per scone

Kcals 128 (528 kj) Protein 3 g Carb 14 g Fat 7 g

Saturated fat 4 g Fibre 1 g

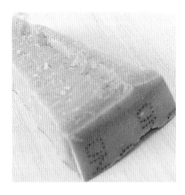

250 g (8 oz) self-raising flour

75 g (3 oz) unsalted butter

4 tablespoons freshly grated Parmesan cheese

3 tablespoons chopped mixed herbs, e.g., oregano and chives

1 egg, beaten

3 tablespoons buttermilk

Roasted Pepper and Tomato Soup (*see page 59*), to serve

1 Sift the flour into a large bowl, add the butter and rub in with the fingertips until the mixture resembles fine breadcrumbs. Add 3 tablespoons of the Parmesan and the herbs and stir together.

2 Beat together the egg and the buttermilk, then using a knife or fork, lightly stir into the dry ingredients to form a dough.

3 Shape the dough into a round roughly 2.5 cm (1 inch) thick, then press out 12 rounds with a 5-cm (2-inch) plain cutter.

4 Place the rounds on a lightly floured baking sheet and sprinkle over the remaining Parmesan. Cook in a preheated oven, 220°C (425°F), Gas Mark 7, for 10–12 minutes until golden and well risen. Serve with roasted pepper and tomato soup. These scones are best eaten on the same day.

CHILLI NAANS
WITH ONION

makes 8
preparation time 5 minutes, plus resting
cooking time 5 minutes

nutritional values per naan
Kcals 136 (561 kj) Protein 3 g Carb 26 g Fat 3 g
Saturated fat 0 g Fibre 1 g

---

250 g (8 oz) self-raising flour, sifted
1 teaspoon cumin seeds
2 teaspoons dried chilli flakes
pinch of salt
2 tablespoons low-fat yogurt
8 tablespoons warm water
2 tablespoons olive oil
1 onion, finely sliced
Chicken Curry with Baby Spinach (*see page 94*), to serve

1 Mix together the flour, cumin seeds, chilli flakes and salt in a large bowl. Combine the yogurt and measurement water and stir into the flour to form a soft dough. Turn the dough out on a lightly floured surface and knead for about a minute until soft and smooth, then cover and rest for 1 hour.

2 Meanwhile, heat half the oil in a small frying pan, add the onion and fry until golden and softened.

3 When the dough has rested, place a thick baking sheet under a high grill. Divide the dough into 8 pieces and roll each out into an oval about 20 cm (8 inches) long and 2.5 cm (1 inch) thick. Brush the tops with the remaining oil.

4 Place 2 naans on the hot baking sheet and cook under the grill for 30 seconds, then turn them over, sprinkle over some of the onion and continue to cook for 20–30 seconds until they are beginning to brown and puff up. Remove and keep them warm while you cook the remaining naans.

5 When all the naans are cooked, serve with chicken curry with baby spinach.

OLIVE AND HALOUMI
BREAD

serves 12

preparation time 15 minutes, plus rising

cooking time 25 minutes

nutritional values per serving

Kcals 189 (780 kj) Protein 7 g Carb 32 g Fat 5 g

Saturated fat 1 g Fibre 2 g

---

500 g (1 lb) strong plain flour, plus extra for sifting

7-g (¼-oz) sachet fast-action dried yeast

pinch of salt

2 tablespoons olive oil

300 ml (½ pint) warm water

1 onion, thinly sliced

100 g (3½ oz) pitted olives

75 g (3 oz) haloumi cheese, chopped

2 tablespoons chopped parsley

to serve

Parma ham and sun-blush tomatoes (optional)

Roasted Pepper and Tomato Soup (*see page 59*) (optional)

1 Place the flour, yeast and salt in a large bowl. Combine half the oil with the measurement water and stir into the flour to form a dough.

2 Turn the dough out on a lightly floured surface and knead for 5 minutes until smooth and elastic. Place in a lightly oiled bowl, cover with a damp cloth and set aside in a warm place for about 1 hour until doubled in size.

3 Meanwhile, heat the remaining oil in a frying pan, add the onion and fry for 7–8 minutes until softened and golden. Leave to cool.

4 Turn the risen dough out on the floured surface and add the remaining ingredients, including the onion, kneading it into the dough. Shape into an oval, place on a lightly floured baking sheet and leave to rise for 1 hour.

5 When the loaf has risen, slash a few cuts in the top, sift over a little flour, then bake in a preheated oven, 220°C (425°F), Gas Mark 7, for about 25 minutes until hollow-sounding when tapped. Transfer to a wire rack to cool. Serve with Parma ham and sun-blush tomatoes or roasted red pepper soup, if desired. This bread may be stored for up to 2 days in an airtight container.

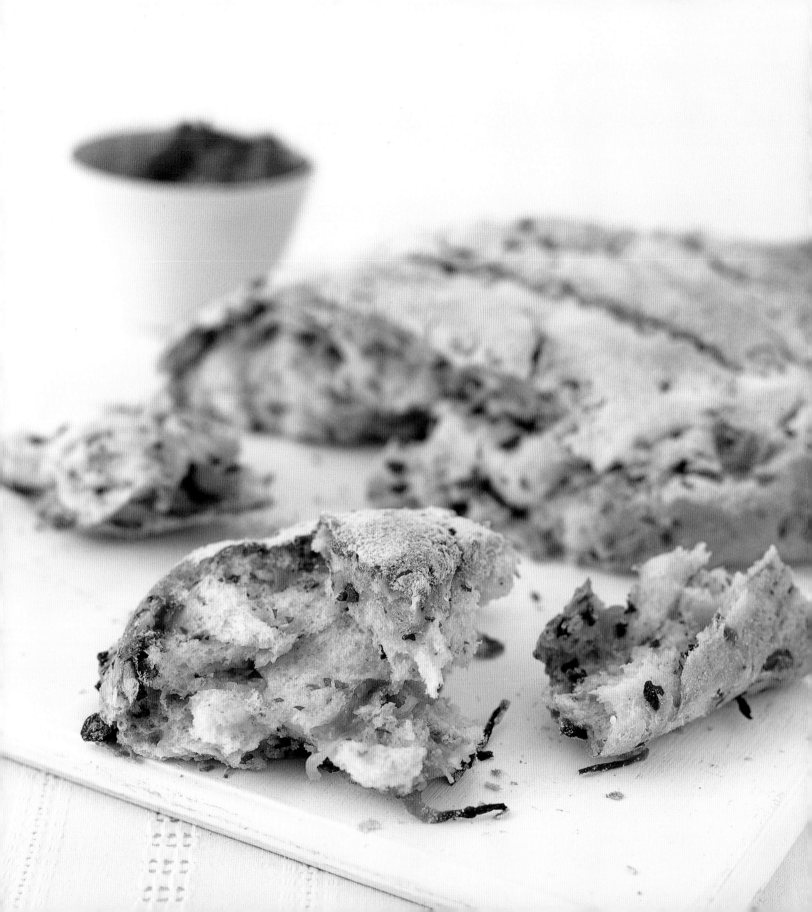

PARMESAN-TOPPED
CHEESY NIBBLES

makes 30

preparation time 10 minutes, plus chilling

cooking time 12 minutes

nutritional values per nibble

Kcals 35 (144 kj) Protein 1 g Carb 3 g Fat 2 g

Saturated fat 1 g Fibre 0 g

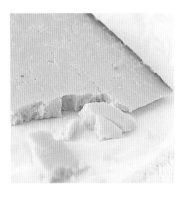

125 g (4 oz) plain flour, sifted

½ teaspoon dried mustard powder

**50 g (2 oz) unsalted butter, softened, or
polyunsaturated margarine**

2 tablespoons light crème fraîche

1 egg yolk

3 tablespoons grated mature Cheddar cheese

1 tablespoon poppy seeds or sesame seeds

milk, for brushing

1 tablespoon freshly grated Parmesan cheese

1 Place all the ingredients, except the milk and Parmesan, in a food processor and process for a few seconds until combined.

2 Turn the mixture out on a lightly floured surface and bring it together to form a dough. Gently roll the dough into a sausage shape about 5 cm (2 inches) in diameter. Wrap in foil then chill for about 30 minutes.

3 Slice the sausage into 30 rounds, place them on nonstick baking sheets and brush with a little milk. Sprinkle over the Parmesan, then cook in a preheated oven, 200°C (400°F), Gas Mark 6, for 10–12 minutes until golden.

4 Transfer to a wire rack to cool and become crisp, then store in an airtight container until required. Serve with drinks. These nibbles may be stored for up to 2 days in an airtight container.

BIG SAVOURY
MUFFINS

makes 12

preparation time 5 minutes

cooking time 25 minutes

nutritional values per muffin

Kcals 147 (607 kj) Protein 3 g Carb 16 g Fat 8 g

Saturated fat 2 g Fibre 1 g

250 g (8 oz) self-raising flour

1 teaspoon baking powder

½ teaspoon bicarbonate of soda

pinch of salt

2 bacon rashers, grilled and chopped

3 spring onions, sliced

8 olives, pitted and roughly chopped

1 tablespoon chopped parsley

50 g (2 oz) Cheddar cheese, grated

6 tablespoons olive oil

125 ml (4 fl oz) semi-skimmed milk

pepper

polyunsaturated margarine, to serve

1 Sift together the flour, baking powder, bicarbonate of soda and salt into a large bowl. Add the bacon, spring onions, olives, parsley and Cheddar and stir together. Season with pepper

2 Mix together the oil and milk and lightly stir into the flour mixture to give a slightly lumpy mixture.

3 Spoon the mixture into a 12-cup muffin tin lined with muffin cases and bake in a preheated oven, 190°C (375°F), Gas Mark 5, for 20–25 minutes until golden and risen. Carefully lift the cases from the tin and transfer to a wire rack to cool.

4 Serve split in half and spread with some polyunsaturated margarine. These muffins are best eaten on the same day.

SUN-DRIED TOMATO
AND PESTO ROLLS

makes 12

preparation time 10 minutes, plus rising

cooking time 20 minutes

nutritional values per roll

Kcals 193 (797 kj) Protein 6 g Carb 32 g Fat 5 g

Saturated fat 1 g Fibre 1 g

7-g (¼-oz) sachet fast-action dried yeast

500 g (1 lb) strong plain flour

good pinch of salt

1 tablespoon olive oil

4 tablespoons ready-made pesto

18 sun-dried tomatoes, roughly chopped

250 ml (8 fl oz) tepid water

a little beaten egg

25 g (1 oz) sunflower seeds

soup, to serve

1 Sift together the yeast, flour and salt into a medium bowl. Make a well in the centre. Mix the oil, pesto and tomatoes into the measurement water, then pour into the well and gradually mix into the flour mixture to form a dough.

2 Turn out on a lightly floured surface and knead for 5 minutes until smooth and elastic. Place in a lightly oiled bowl, cover with a damp cloth and set aside in a warm place for about 1 hour until doubled in size.

3 Turn the risen dough out on the floured surface, knead again for a few minutes, then divide into 12 pieces. Shape into rolls, place on a lightly floured baking sheet, then cover and leave to double in size again.

4 When the rolls have risen, brush the tops with a little beaten egg, then sprinkle over the sunflower seeds. Bake in a preheated oven, 220°C (425°F), Gas Mark 7, for about 20 minutes until golden and hollow-sounding when tapped. Transfer to a wire rack to cool. Serve with any of the soups in this book. These rolls may be stored for up to 2 days in an airtight container.

APPLE, CHEESE
AND NUT LOAF

serves 4

preparation time 10 minutes

cooking time 40 minutes

nutritional values per serving

Kcals 275 (1135 kj) Protein 9 g Carb 32 g Fat 13 g

Saturated fat 5 g Fibre 3 g

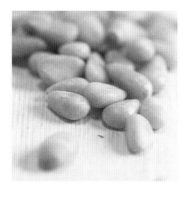

200 g (7 oz) self-raising flour

250 g (8 oz) self-raising wholemeal flour

40 g (1½ oz) unsalted butter, cut into small pieces

1 large eating apple, peeled, cored and finely chopped

150 g (5 oz) feta cheese, crumbled

75 g (3 oz) pine nuts, roughly chopped

2 tablespoons chopped parsley

8–10 tablespoons semi-skimmed milk

1 egg yolk, beaten

pepper

1 Sift the flours into a large bowl, adding any bran in the sieve. Add the butter and rub in with the fingertips until the mixture resembles fine breadcrumbs. Season with pepper.

2 Stir in the apple, feta, pine nuts and parsley with a fork and rub in with the fingertips, then mix in enough milk to make a soft dough. Turn the dough out on a lightly floured surface and shape into a round approximately 20 cm (8 inches) in diameter.

3 Brush the top with beaten egg and cut a lattice pattern, then place on a lightly floured baking sheet and bake in a preheated oven, 190°C (375°F), Gas Mark 5, for 35–40 minutes until golden. Turn the loaf over and continue to bake for 5 minutes. Serve warm. This loaf is best eaten on the same day.

INDEX

ACKNOWLEDGEMENTS

Executive Editor: Nicola Hill
Editors: Alice Bowden, Rachel Lawrence
Executive Art Editor: Karen Sawyer
Designer: Miranda Harvey
Senior Production Controller: Manjit Sihra
Photographer: Lis Parsons
Food stylists: David Morgan, Annie Nichols
Props stylist: Rachel Jukes

Special Photography by © Octopus
Publishing Group Limited/Lis Parsons.

Other Photography:
Octopus Publishing Group Limited/Frank
Adam 19, 122, 140; /Gus Filgate 51; /Sandra
Lane 39; /William Lingwood 74; /David
Loftus 86; /Sean Myers 26, 30, 34, 78, 109,
127, 150, 157; /William Reavell 50, 66, 118.

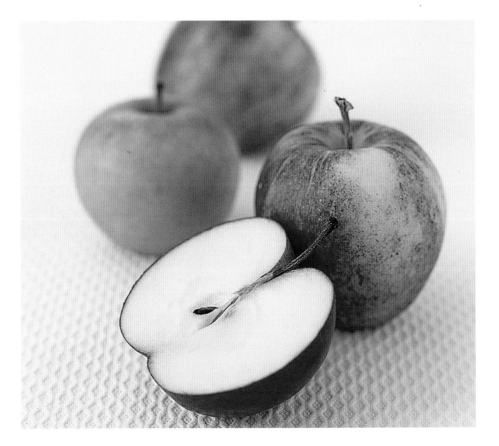